IVF AND JUSTICE

IVF AND JUSTICE

Moral, Social and Legal Issues Related to Human *in vitro* Fertilisation

TERESA IGLESIAS

THE LINACRE CENTRE
FOR HEALTH CARE ETHICS
London 1990

Published by The Linacre Centre,
60 Grove End Road, London NW8 9NH.
© The Linacre Centre, 1990

First published 1990

British Library Cataloguing in Publication Data
Iglesias, Teresa
IVF and Justice: moral, social and legal issues related
to human in vitro fertilisation.
1. Women. Ova. In vitro fertilisation. Ethical aspects.
I. Title   II. Linacre Centre
176

ISBN 0–906561–07–8

Photoset and printed in Great Britain by
Redwood Press Limited, Melksham, Wiltshire

For Martin and Patrick

Contents

Acknowledgements

Six chapters of this book are based on papers already published. Thanks are due to the editors and the publishers of the various journals and books in which these papers appeared for allowing me to reproduce them. The original publications were the following: 'In Vitro Fertilization: The Major Ethical Issues', in *Journal of Medical Ethics*, vol. 10, no. 1, March, 1984, pp. 32–37; 'Social and Ethical Aspects of IVF', in Ian Donald (ed.), *Test-Tube Babies*, Unity Press, London, 1984, pp. 67–94; 'The Concept of "Human Person"', in *Study Guide to 'Euthanasia and Clinical Practice'*, The Linacre Centre, London, 1984, pp. 42–47; *A Basic Ethic for Man's Wellbeing: Conscience and the New Scientific Possibilities*, Booklet Series, World Federation of Doctors who Respect Human Life, Liverpool, 1984; *Artificial Insemination in Vivo and In Vitro: A Report to the European Parliament*, from a hearing held in the European Parliament for the Commission Juridique et des Droits des Citoyens, November 27–29, 1985 (Archives, PE 102.135/8); 'What Kind of Being is the Human Embryo?', in Nigel M de S Cameron (ed.), *Embryos and Ethics: The Warnock Report in Debate*, Rutherford House Books, Edinburgh, 1987, pp. 58–73. There was no opportunity to revise the substance or arguments of these papers, but all of them have undergone stylistic revision. However, the differing styles of reference in the footnotes to the original papers have been retained.

It is not possible to arrive at an adequate judgement concerning the central issues of the beginning of the life of the human being and of its end at death without detailed attention to the empirical facts of our organic human condition, as we now know them (i.e., fertilisation, early embryonic development, brain death, etc.). I am not a scientist; my primary expertise is philosophical. Nevertheless, the need to study empirical facts (biological and technological) has been paramount in my research. My understanding and interpretation of these facts have been checked against the findings of many experts in the various scientific fields. On embryology I have had the opportunity either to correspond or to converse with some authorities, particularly Professor R. G. Edwards, Dr A. McLaren, Dr J. M. W. Slack, Professor J. Lejeune and Dr J. McLean. Some of these scientists share my moral convictions, others do not. Dr C. Pallis, Dr D. W. Evans and my brother Dr J. R. Iglesias, neuropathologist at the Universitätsklinikum Rudolf Virchow, Berlin, have been of great assistance in helping me to understand the physiological facts related to brain death. Dr Peggy Norris, of the Medical Education Trust, has been a constant source of encouragement in my work and always of assistance in providing invaluable information from the Trust archives. I have also profited from extended conversations with colleagues in philosophy, as well as with lawyers and theologians. The questions and comments raised by the audiences who have listened to me and by the nursing and medical students whom I have been teaching, have helped me to crystallise and clarify my thoughts. I thank them all.

Generous financial assistance for this publication was provided by the National University of Ireland, by University College, Dublin, by my former professor, Archbishop Desmond Connell, as well as by donors who wish to remain anonymous.

I am grateful to the Linacre Centre for making the papers available in this form. Mr Luke Gormally, the Director of the Centre, has given unfailingly generous assistance to my work over the years. Dr F. J. Fitzpatrick has spent much time and effort in editing the typescript, and Mrs Agneta Sutton has kindly helped with the proofs. I am most grateful to them all. My colleague at University College, Dublin, Dr P. K. Bastable, has been of invaluable help.

T. I.

Introduction

The *in vitro* conceptus and justice

1. Human *in vitro* fertilization is an issue of justice. This statement may appear surprising. For IVF is commonly regarded as primarily a technological intervention to assist human conception in order to help couples who are infertile. When, in 1978, a baby girl conceived by the *in vitro* technique (the first 'test-tube baby') was born in England, IVF found a great deal of acceptance – as was shown by the natural response by lay people of welcoming Louise Brown into the world. She had been born to parents who could not have conceived otherwise. Why, then, over the last 12 years, has IVF technology given rise to so much public debate, particularly within parliaments? The precise controversy that has taken place would not have arisen if the sole objective of IVF procedures, and the sole result of implementing them, were that of attaining conception from the parents' gametes outside the wife's body and of having the conceptus transferred to her womb, while maintaining respect for the integrity and wellbeing of the individual conceptus.

2. Although the aim of assisting infertile couples to conceive was publicly presented as the overriding objective of the IVF technique, once the human gametes and the early embryo were made available for human handling in the laboratory, other 'therapeutic' and scientific ends were also envisaged and defended by those pioneering the technique. These ends required direct experimentation and destruction of human embryos.[1] They were:

1

- the improvement of the IVF technique itself;
- the study of inherited diseases;
- the detection of genetic abnormalities in the embryo, leading to 'test-tube abortion';[2]
- the use of embryonic tissue for transplantation;
- the scientific study of human embryogenesis, that is to say, 'embryology for its own sake';[3]
- the development of 'safer means of contraception',[4] including the manufacturing of an 'anti-pregnancy vaccine'.[5]

3. There is no doubt that the 1980s will be seen as a decade in which issues related to medico-scientific technology and human generation were the subject of social, moral and legal concern. In most European countries, as well as in America, Australia and elsewhere, some forms of legislation or regulation have been debated and introduced in relation to IVF and allied practices. But the need for further debate and legal provision is strongly felt and demanded.[6] The main issues in the debate have been, and still are,[7] the manner in which the human conceptus generated *in vitro* (i.e., in a glass dish in the laboratory) is to be treated by parents, doctors and scientists, and how ultimately it is to be protected by law. These are fundamental issues of justice, both morally and legally. If this were not so they would not be discussed at length by parliamentarians and by ordinary people.

4. In regard to legislation it must be obvious that before the IVF technique was developed, the law could not have been concerned with the possibility that a human being might be generated and begin to exist outside the human body in a laboratory, and never be transferred to a womb. Nevertheless, in the nineteenth century legal provision had been made for the protection of the embryonic human being, conceived naturally *in vivo*, within the body of a woman.

5. Arguably, some of these provisions could be applied by courts to the conceptus transferred to the womb after external *in vitro* conception. English law, for example, makes provision in the Offences against the Persons Act, 1861, to prevent a deliberate 'miscarriage of any woman' (a phrase which

2

occurs in both section 58 and section 59 of that Act). But since the *in vitro* conceptus is not a being 'carried' by any woman, there is no possibility of 'miscarriage'. Similarly, the provisions made in the Infant Life (Preservation) Act, 1929, protect the child only 'before it has an existence independent of its mother'. The *in vitro* conceptus is already independent of its mother, and could even be generated without reference to a mother at all. Some lawyers would defend the view that the spirit of the law, if rightly interpreted, protects the conceptus from the time of its origin. (It must be noted that the laws decriminalising induced abortion did not abrogate the 1861 and 1929 Acts but permitted abortion only in some established cases of conflict of interest between the wishes of the mother and the life of the child.) It is true that practices and precedents of established law could be invoked for protection of the *in vitro* conceptus. This would happen in practice in most contexts if the moral attitudes prevalent in our society were in continuity with those attitudes which permitted the framing of older laws to protect the intra-uterine life of the human being from conception. But we have now reached a point at which such a continuity has been partially broken. Moral attitudes enshrined in the law to protect the total life-span of the human being are being opposed and abandoned.

6. The law, and the traditional ethic which it enshrined, were expressions of a moral perspective which recognised the supreme worth of the individual human being. The established law on these matters treated the conceptus as a human entity, a being falling within the category of human beings (people), that is, as a human being in embryonic form deserving, like every other human being, to have its life preserved, a being therefore not outside the application of human justice. Today attempts are made to place the human *in vitro* conceptus outside the realm of justice, by claiming that it is not a being entitled to protection of its life and to human respect. These attempts are designed to make it seem to be a being outside the human fraternity, beyond the human pale.

7. What is really at stake here is the understanding of who we are: What is it to be human? What are the roots of our human

identity? What are the foundations of man's biological nature? Is our embryonic beginning to be denied? Has it not true reality and significance? What are the human bonds constituting the human family? Do parentage, kinship and descent cease to be relevant to our human identity? What is it that demarcates human beings from things, from other animals and from God? What does it mean to say that I am bodily, and that in a true sense I *am* my body? How can I accept that had I been an *in vitro* conceptus, my embryonic existence would have been truly outside the realm of humanity, that it would have been of a quite distinct nature from the nature I have now, and so I would not have deserved protection and respect? Do we or do we not all share our embodied humanity? Are we not all *equally* human? Where does *human* equality rest?

8. Fundamental claims of justice emerge from the nature of what we are. This truth grounds the general perspective from which this book is written. The most basic form of justice may be called 'attributive',[8] since it recognises and attributes to beings what they are and what they can claim to be and become, and hence it sets conditions and provisions for those claims to be realised. This is the form of justice enshrined in every law as its 'moral norm'; the law does, and must, distinguish between human beings and other entities and treat the various beings accordingly. Debates about the dignity of our shared humanity, and the respect each one of us deserves as a human being, morally and legally, are to be settled not on the basis of a religious doctrine but on the basis of what is naturally knowable about what we truly are. It is this which determines justice and which is the only acceptable standard for responsible discussion of the respect owed to human beings. The reasons which a religious person, as a person of conscience, might advance for taking up a position on this matter are not different in kind from the reasons which should guide the conscience of those who profess no religion at all. Our shared humanity is a fact. It is to be hoped that responsible people will come to substantial general agreement that the notion of a 'lesser humanity' or of a 'lesser human being' is untenable; but if they do not, such differences as they have will be within a common content and structure of reasoning: they will be

differences on a matter of justice. Some human beings will enjoy the protection of justice themselves, while seeking, for their own advantage, to bring it about that others will not.

9. Most of the chapters in this book were written during a period of four years (1982–1986) when I had to consider in some depth the moral issues raised by IVF. I was then Research Officer at the Linacre Centre for Health Care Ethics, London. My research resulted in various papers which were first delivered at conferences and later published. Most of these papers are collected in this volume. Chapter Six, 'Death and the Beginning of Life', although based on research carried out in those years, has been written recently and is published here for the first time. The articles have been revised in order to avoid unnecessary repetition. Originally a certain amount of repetition was inevitable, given that the various articles record lectures on various aspects of the same topics, delivered to different audiences. Chapter Seven, because it has the character of a report made to a legislative body, has been altered only very slightly. Since 1986 some technological developments have occurred in relation to IVF, for example the freezing of human ova; also, further evidence has come to light concerning the results of the procedure and the dangers which it involves.[9] Nevertheless the moral, social and legal issues raised remain the same. The necessary revisions, therefore, have not been great.

10. The central theme running through the book, which was brought to the fore by IVF technology, is that of the nature of the human conceptus and the moral claims that it makes upon us. But this is an issue closely related to other major social concerns, such as the nature of scientific endeavour, the role of technology in medicine and the nature of medicine itself. Are scientists to seek knowledge, engage in research, do whatever is technically possible, independently of the moral obligation they have to serve the true end of their endeavour, which should ultimately be the promotion of the well-being of each and every human being? Can medicine remain the healing art when the most fundamental Hippocratic commands, 'Do not harm' and 'Benefit the sick', have been abandoned as absolute

5

norms in dealing with each and every patient, and when respect for human life from conception no longer holds? These questions are treated in the first two chapters, in which IVF technology is presented and discussed in its medico-scientific setting. The issue of research is said to be central to IVF technology, and in this context a fundamental moral question arises: what are the lawful and best reasearch approaches to helping those who are infertile? The focus of moral difficulty here is the fate of the embryonic beings that are brought into existence in laboratories (either as a necessary part of an IVF process to benefit an infertile couple, or otherwise for research purposes) and which do not belong to the 'elite group' of embryos that are nurtured, maternally, to birth. The question arises: Does the IVF technique assist infertile couples only at the cost of committing grave injustice against many new human beings? The essential issue here is not research but *lawful* research, not IVF as such but whether in fact it is possible to have IVF without the presence of grave injustice. In this book, the answer given is that in practice it is not possible (Chapters One and Two). In Chapter Two attention is also paid to the socio-moral problem related to the abandonment of truth in social relations, particularly in relations of parentage: What possible norm of justice can be invoked to defend the view that (e.g.) a child should be prevented from knowing who his genetic parents are?

11. Chapters Three, Four and Five complement each other in the attempt to present a picture of the human and personal nature of the conceptus. There is no doubt that the most crucial issue which has come to the fore in the controversy concerning IVF is: What is the status of the fertilised ovum, the *in vitro* conceptus? Is it a new individual, a human being, a human person, 'one of us'?; Is it *me* at the earliest moments of *my* life? Some have defended the idea that the early human conceptus 'should be treated as a thing',[10] so that the concept of property-ownership would become applicable to it. Others would say that the human conceptus falls neither within the category of thing or 'product', nor within the category of person, 'but in some other category altogether'. To consider the *in vitro* conceptus as either a thing or a human being is, it is

alleged, to accept 'a false dichotomy';[11] on this view *in vitro* conceptuses deserve 'some' protection, but not necessarily an absolute protection against being destroyed. (Obviously the meaning and content of the words 'some protection' must be empty if we consider each conceptus individually – and that is the only way it can be considered – for what would it mean to say that I have 'some' protection in law but not protection against being destroyed?) Thus the debate rests today on the issue of whether the human conceptus is ontologically (i.e., in its being and nature), morally and legally an entity falling within the category of (a) a person, 'one of us', in his or her embryonic stage; or (b) a thing, a piece of property, which can be destroyed, bought and sold; or (c) an 'in-between' entity of a type yet to be determined.

12. Much of the controversy on this topic has been conducted in the context of contemporary biological knowledge of fertilisation and of the early days of embryonic development. Thus great attention has been focused on the 14th day of life, before which, some argue, there is either (i) no embryonic individual at all but only a living mass, a 'cluster of human cells', or (ii) an embryonic being that is human but not of a personal nature. My conviction, for which I argue in this book, is that the humanity of the early human conceptus, ontologically, morally and legally must be upheld; the human conceptus is 'one of us', or, to put it in other words, the human conceptus falls within the category of *people in the early stages of their lives*; by 'people' is meant what we ordinarily call human beings and human persons. The arguments defending this position in the central chapters of this book are made from various perspectives.

13. The first perspective may be regarded as scientific. In view of the known biological facts of early human embryonic development, biologists classify the human embryo as a living being (not as a mere 'cluster of cells') belonging to the human species and formed at fertilisation (sharing this form of origin with all other mammalian animal embryos). Hence biologists talk of the early human embryo (the zygote) as 'the beginning of the human individual' or as 'the beginning of human

7

development'. Neither the unity and individuality of the embryo (i.e., the fact that it is one embryo physically and functionally) nor the continuity of its development is ever questioned by biologists; rather these are facts observed, recognised and acknowledged, facts involving the working of mechanisms which scientists attempt to understand and account for. Our bodily organic existence begins at fertilisation (conception). This is a fact, not a theory. Even Dr R. G. Edwards testifies to it: 'Human life begins in the obscurity of the oviducts, virtually inaccessible to observation, as the fusion of spermatozoon and egg results in the production of an embryo.'[12] He has also been reported to have said about Louise Brown: 'The last time I saw her, she was just eight cells in a test-tube. She was beautiful then and she's still beautiful now.'[13] The fact that the embryo may divide and give rise to identical twins, or even the fact that scientists by technical manipulation may disaggregate and aggregate the cells of early embryos, does not alter the fact that *the natural norm* is that a single human being begins at fertilisation.

14. From a philosophical perspective it should be clear that if there is a continuity of development in the embryo (i.e. a development from zygote to embryo to fetus to infant), as in fact there is, that continuity points to the embryo's being one and the same entity in its development; it develops by its own immanent internal power, and eventually it becomes the fully developed human being. Hence the embryo must be said to possess at least the *potential* to become the human adult. But this is often interpreted as meaning that the embryo has 'humanity claims' upon us only because of what it will become in the future, and not in virtue of what it is now. This is to acknowledge only half the truth of what 'potentiality' means. Potentiality resides in an actual power, in something actually present in the embryo, making it the kind of being it is now, constituting it as *this kind* of entity now; the embryo actually has a power (a 'constitutional power', as I call it) in virtue of which it becomes the adult. Thus, the embryo has claims of respect upon us because of what it is now as well as what it will be. In the words of Leon Kass: 'In the blastocyst, even in the zygote, we face a mysterious and awesome power, a power

8

governed by an immanent plan that may produce an indisputably and fully human being. It deserves our respect ... because of what it is now *and* prospectively'.[14] The humanity of the embryo resides in its organic physical make-up, endowed as it is with the power of being human now, as an embryo, and of becoming an adult. It is in our bodily make-up that our humanity is totally given. I thus argue for an affirmative answer to the question: Does the beginning and the end of the organic bodily life of a human being constitute the beginning and the end of his or her human life?

15. I maintain, then, that the nature of the embryo is indisputably human, that is, that the human embryo is a human being in his or her embryonic stage of existence. But I go on to argue also that there are no grounds for dividing the members of the human family into persons and non-persons. The word 'person', and even the terms 'human being' and 'people', may sound somewhat unusual when applied to a human conceptus; for we do not talk to human conceptuses, nor do they count on population registers; their 'social existence' has not yet started. But the fundamental issue is not whether the term 'person' (or other terms) should always be used for embryos or not; what is at stake is their true identity, and whether we can acknowledge embryos as human beings whose human nature or identity is already established at that very early stage. Because the organic bodily constitution of the conceptus is entirely human, because it clearly possesses an immanent power of remaining human, of growing and of eventually becoming an adult, there must be a subject to which this bodily constitution and this power belong. And as the power that the embryo manifests is that of becoming an adult person, it must be said that the embryo possesses this 'personal' power, that it is constituted by this power, and hence that the embryo must be recognised as a personal subject, that is, an entity endowed with a personal nature.

16. Although some philosophers would not oppose the essential points in the claims just made, others would argue that there are difficulties to be faced which prevent us from accepting the humanity of the embryo, that is, from recognising the

9

embryo as 'one of us'. The difficulties appear to centre on the issues of identical twinning and embryo recombination. It is alleged that the early embryo can divide to form (e.g.) identical twins, or that two distinct embryos can somehow fuse to form a single one; and it is thought that this latter occurrence – the fusion of two embryos into one – not only occurs in nature but may be brought about in the laboratory. If this is the case, then, it is claimed, the embryo in its early stages cannot be regarded as an 'individual', that is, as a single human and personal being; it cannot be an individual in the sense of one human and personal subject which is indivisible as a subject and continues to be that subject throughout organic development. An individual which is divisible, it is assumed, cannot remain an individual entity throughout change. Hence the individual does not have continuity of existence as a subject; in fact it is not a subject at all, for it cannot be one and the same subject throughout the change. Many would identify the human personal subject with an 'immortal soul' and then argue that if the embryo is divisible, it is not a human individual subject, is hence without a human soul; that it is therefore in no sense 'one of us' and consequently does not deserve protection of its life or the kind of respect that we deserve.

17. It is important to note that if these difficulties appear substantial, it is because they are set in a context in which the larger and most fundamental question, 'What is it to be human?', is not asked, and in which the fact that our humanity is given in our bodily condition is totally dismissed and lost sight of. In this book I have primarily attempted to focus on the difficulties as they are raised. In this respect there is no doubt that many of the alleged 'difficulties' emerge in relation to a particular conception (philosophical and theological) of the 'soul'. Hence a good philosophy and a good theology of the soul is what is required to deal properly with those difficulties. In the present volume such a thorough analysis of the nature of the soul is not provided; but basic points and insights to dispel current misconceptions are given (see Chapter Five, paras. 34–41).

18. Many authors would claim that these difficulties are not primarily of a philosophical nature but are rather fundamentally biological, that is, based on the biological facts as we know them today. In this context my contribution here is to provide a framework which enables us to think of the alleged difficulties of twinning and recombination as really 'non-difficulties', for they can be shown to arise from a limited perspective which ignores the fact that the early embryo is a living being, a living whole, and not a mere conglomeration of cells. The human conceptus, like the embryo of any other animal, is an entity which falls, in biological terms, under the category of living being: that is, the conceptus has a physical organic constitution, powers and functions proper to a living being. Biologically, each living being is one, a whole and individual being from generation to death, and it does not cease to be *that* one, and *that* individual, unless through death (see Chapter Five, paras. 23–27). A living being as a whole does not turn into two or more living beings, nor into another living being; nor does it fuse with one or other living being to become a new one. But it is the case that parts or fragments of the living being (be they molecules, cells or tissues) can be detached or cut off from it and added to other beings. Divisions and recombinations of embryonic *cells* can certainly be brought about in the laboratory, but not divisions and recombinations of *embryos themselves as wholes*. A living being itself as a whole does not divide or recombine. Thus I hold that 'Every living being is individual, that is, organically individuated in all its dimensions from its generation (whether brought about sexually or asexually) to its death'.

19. I draw attention to the relationship between truths of philosophy and truths of Christian faith in relation to the human conceptus, because for many audiences who heard or read the various papers reproduced here this was an important issue. The main point here is that truths of faith do not ultimately rest on evidence (or the lack of it) provided by theories, whether scientific or philosophical (see Chapter Five, paras. 28–34).

11

20. In Chapter Six I am concerned with the idea that it is important that our understanding of the beginning of a human life should cohere in every way with our understanding of death, its ending. This means posing the question: What is the criterion enabling me to judge 'This human organism is dead; it is no longer a bodily person, no longer a human personal being, no longer a patient, but a corpse'? This question is independent of the moral problem of euthanasia and of deciding which means of prolonging the lives of human beings are justified and which are not, although the way we answer the question can make a contribution to decision-making on these issues. The fundamental point of Chapter Six is to show that 'the medical profession is, and has always been, of the view and practice that a patient is, without qualification, the human bodily being still alive; furthermore, the new knowledge gained which permits us to understand death as 'brain death' ratifies this vision and practice' (para. 6).

21. What is good and necessary legislation concerning IVF? The answer to this question is given in Chapter Seven, in the form of recommendations which I put to legislators in the European Parliament. The recommendations can be substantially summed up in this one: 'Laws are about establishing and implementing *principles of justice*. One of these principles, enshrined in our laws, is that the human being is not property, not chattel. He or she cannot be bought and sold. To abolish this principle from present legal frameworks, and to introduce its opposite, is to accept and legalise a new form of slavery, and so to deny the most fundamental requirements of a just society' (Chapter Seven, para.45.(3)).

22. Before this book went to press the British Parliament approved a law which permits scientific research involving harmful and destructive experimentation on human embryos, generated *in vitro*, up to the 14th day of their existence (and within a period not greater than five years if embryos are stored). The main recommendations made by the majority of members of the Warnock Committee in their Report, which was submitted to the Government in 1984, have constituted

the basis of the present law. There are a few comments that I want to make concerning this new legislation and its relation to justice.

(i) *Parliament has enacted a law whereby some human beings are legally reduced to the status of things.* Legally, in Britain, the early human embryo *in vitro* (and, by implication, every human being in his or her early embryonic form) has been reduced to the status of a thing, i.e., a useful and disposable asset. Norms of justice are not applicable to things; we design these norms to govern relationships among human beings only. Now, embryonic human beings are by law declared to be outside the realm of humanity. Legally, human embryos can now be generated, stored, bought, sold, chemically used, dissected, disposed of. This is approved in view of the 'good consequences' (i.e. benefits – of 'therapeutic' or scientific nature) that the procedures bring about for other human beings. This is the kind of consequentialist ethical outlook which leads to the reduction of some human beings to the status of useful things, serving as means to benefit other human beings.

Consequentialism has a long history. It is, of course, the underlying logic of the 'slavery ethic'. There is no doubt that embryonic human beings and unborn children are the 'slaves' of our age; they may be used or disposed of, given certain 'necessities' for those who are 'full humans' and have the power to exclude others legally from humanity and destroy them. Our civilisation has legally adopted embryocide and feticide, while infanticide – not being yet legal – is openly advocated. In ancient times three categories of human beings were identified as 'lesser humans', namely, slaves, women and children. It was only in the first half of the last century that slavery was legally abolished. In recent decades the feminist movement has made it socially unacceptable in certain parts of the world to regard women as a 'lesser kind' of human being. 'Equality for women' and 'women's rights' unfortunately are not everywhere defended and implemented. Yet, paradoxically, many men and women in our time consider that the humanity of children and of the unborn is still to be governed by the slavery ethic. Justice for the unborn is still on the waiting list.

13

(ii) *Parliament has enacted a law which imposes a duty to destroy or dispose of human life*. A feature of the new British law concerns the fact that it does not only permit harmful and destructive experimentation on human embryos up to the 14th day of their existence; the law is a command to destroy or 'dispose of' the embryo or to 'allow [it] to perish' before it has reached the 15th day. To kill now becomes mandatory, thus the law now does not only permit us to deliberately harm some individual human beings, but makes it a duty. The meaning of justice has been turned upside down.

(iii) *Parliament has established expedient 'legal control' but not fundamental justice*. There is a radical departure, in the present British legislation, from a previous law designed to protect every human being from the time of his or her conception. In the process of public debate in Britain it has become clear that the majority of the Warnock Committee, and of those supporting them, were not concerned with examining the moral nature of this departure and whether it could be justified in view of principles of justice. Rather their main concern was 'controlling' the practices which scientists and doctors were *already* engaged in, involving destructive use of human embryos. Hence the major concern (as stated in the Report and recently reiterated by Baroness Warnock) was to offer a framework of 'legal control' for those practices in order to 'allay public anxiety'. This, it has been said, is a 'triumph for the law',[15] ensuring that doctors and scientists have a limit imposed on their destructive experimentation on human subjects beyond which they cannot go, namely, the 14th day. In reality it is a pragmatic measure. Justice has been ignored.

(iv) *Parliament has ratified laws which abolish the absolute right to justice of every individual human being*. Scientific and medical embryocide is not logically and morally disconnected from fetiscide. The law of 1967 permitting induced abortion introduced a principle which abolished the application of the norms of justice for every human being. The new law ratifies this abolition. (By 'justice' I mean here what I meant above, something very basic: protecting individual human beings from intentional harm.) Morally and legally, there are only two possible alternative ways of regarding the human being; either he is justly respected or he is not; either he is recognised

14

to have intrinsic worth or he is not; either he is to be regarded as a chattel to be used and ultimately disposed of for the benefit of others, or he is not. In other words either a legal system upholds justice for the individual or it does not. Any legal system, as any moral theory and moral practice, necessarily falls under one of these alternatives; there is no possible compromise.

The issue of justice for the concrete individual is the crucial issue of law and human relationships. In fact the whole history of moral and political philosophy could be viewed from this perspective. This is a point which has been summed up in a masterly fashion by G. E. M. Anscombe. She does so in a footnote to her influential paper on 'Modern Moral Philosophy'. While making particular reference to the British tradition in morals, the footnote is of universal significance in the criticism of consequentialist thought and practice. Here it is:

> Oxford Objectivists, of course, distinguish between 'consequences' and 'intrinsic values' and so produce a misleading appearance of not being consequentialists. But they do not hold – and Ross explicitly denies – that the gravity of, e.g., procuring the condemnation of the innocent is such that it cannot be outweighed by, e.g., national interest. Hence their distinction is of no importance. (*Collected Philosophical Papers*, Volume III, p. 33.)

23. In dealing with important public matters, as with everyday ones, may truth be our only authority.

Teresa Iglesias

15

1

A basic ethic for man's well-being: conscience and the new scientific possibilities

I. Conscience and science

1. Every one of us, every human person, should live according to his or her conscience and never shrink from the responsibility of being a thoroughly conscientious person. This is, in a nutshell, 'the basic ethic for man's well-being' which I intend to consider. Let me call this ethic, for our present purposes, 'a Hippocratic ethic'.

The terms 'science' and 'conscience' aptly indicate the context in which my considerations will be set. For the most fundamental moral problems with which we are confronted – and to which we have to respond as conscientious persons – arise from the new scientific possibilities currently affecting the world of medicine.

2. The word 'ethics' primarily refers to a science, that is, to the systematic study of general principles which govern man's moral life. It is, indeed, crucially important for the conscientious person to be well informed ethically; it is important for him to dwell on and consider that kind of ethical reflection, study and tradition which has exercised other great minds seeking understanding, systematisation and moral wisdom. Nevertheless the individual person may find himself or herself – as in fact most of us do – in an environment characterised by public ethical controversy, ethical doubt, ethical inadequacy, even public ethical ignorance. Yet the presence of that public controversy, doubt and ignorance does not remove from the individual person the obligation to be

thoroughly conscientious in all the *particular* and *existential* circumstances of his life. Every individual doctor now lives in an environment in which he must exercise his personal conscience in relation to science, that is, in which he must respond conscientiously to the new medico-scientific possibilities. This awesome and unavoidable responsibility, one which carries enormous social significance and repercussions, is with every one of us, and particularly with every member of the medical and other health-care professions.

3. I take for granted – and as an obvious premise in my argument – that the human person possesses a *natural tendency* (that is, a tendency which is, in part, constitutive of his or her being) towards truth and goodness. This natural tendency develops with conscious life, and becomes an *imperative* awareness of what is true and what is good. In other words, in recognising what is truly good, what is truly of value, we feel compelled to act on our knowledge. A judgement of moral truth, that is, a judgement of value (of right and wrong, of good and evil) is experienced by the person as a judgement of duty and so as something impelling him to act. Thus the *conscientious person* is an *acting person*. He seeks to determine what is truly good and to act accordingly. This judgement of value and this experience of being impelled to action express the dynamism of our consciences, what we might also call the 'conscientious unity', in ourselves, of what is true and of what we are obliged to do.

This is illustrated by the fact that when a norm or directive is presented to us by our own conscience as true there is no stress or resentment in our convictions and our autonomy for action. Yet, by contrast, there is stress and resistance and weakness of conviction when such a norm or directive is presented from outside – from some external authority, for instance – simply as a duty. It is clear that to respond to this inner personal moral dynamism which is our conscience, that is, *to be a conscientious person*, is the fundamental principle of an ethic which is orientated to our general well-being. For it responds to our moral nature without distorting it, and hence without the acceptance of disorder into our lives. Yes, it is our

17

moral nature to have to strive always to become, and to continue to be, fully conscientious persons.[1]

4. Two related aspects of a conscientious person deserve to be stressed here. They could be described as follows: (i) a conscientious person must be *well-affected*; (ii) a conscientious person must be *well-informed*. By being 'well-affected' I mean being 'humanly affected' by the situation, or being 'fully human or full of human feeling'; perceiving with great human-ness the kinds of concrete situations and persons to which we have to respond; really to feel 'as a human being', as we so often put it. There is a great danger of being too abstract; there is a danger – the consequences of which are experienced by many – of looking at concrete problems and concrete human beings as general cases, as states of affairs, as cogs in machines or stages reached in scientific developments and enterprises, as diseases to be cured or dismissed, as problems to be solved. The generalisations, 'scienticisms', euphemisms and, in general, the abstract character of much current debate are symptoms of this distance from reality; we find, for example, that the human embryo is described simply as 'human tissue', human individual care and attention as 'clinical management', particular human persons as 'human life' (and as 'a continuous process without beginning or end'); and the environment in which a human being may begin to exist and develop is dismissed as almost of no significance. Let me give you an example. Professor Carl Wood (one of the pioneers in developing the techniques of human *in vitro* fertilisation in Australia) has written:

> At one stage . . . the team [tried] fertilisation of a human egg and sperm cell, and embryo growth, in the sheep. After collecting a mature egg from the patient, we placed it and sperm cells from her husband in the sheep oviduct . . . But whereas the sperm cells survived in this environment, we were unable to find any trace of the egg. In some ways we were relieved at the failure of this experiment as it may have been difficult to convince the community that the sheep was an appropriate place for human fertilisation and embryo development.[2]

To be human – to accept, acknowledge, know, describe, feel and respond adequately to our humanness – is fundamental to the conscientious person in order to respond with adequate conscientious decisions to concrete situations. People who are really humane, and who have not distanced themselves from the human condition in the concrete, in all its dimensions, surely could not demand that unborn children, and thousands of embryos, be destroyed. It is well known that when it comes to decisions which touch on basic human values, and particularly to decisions of life and death, the attitudes of general practitioners who are always dealing with 'their patients' are strikingly different from the attitudes of scientists, medical researchers, or those merely interested in medical advances.[3] If, then, we are to be well-affected persons, we need to have a lively awareness of the concrete realities, both overall and in their different dimensions. An adequate response necessarily requires adequate knowledge, and this demands of the conscientious person, who should be able to 'see all sides', that he is fully engaged in the situation, that is, that he be well-affected and well-informed. In facing the problems that currently confront us, the need to know all the facts – the actual procedures, accurate scientific truths and possibilities – is crucial both for our evaluations and for determining what we are to do. It is obvious that we cannot respond adequately to a situation if we do not know what the situation actually is. Because this is obvious it requires no further elaboration. Yet, sadly, accurate knowledge of the facts is commonly absent in public debate and decision. But as individuals we cannot succumb to this ignorance in our own conscientious evaluations. I shall illustrate this later with an example (Part IV below). Let me now move to considerations of the new medico-scientific possibilities and to some of the problems to which they give rise.

5. There are many ways in which new scientific discoveries and techniques have enhanced our ability to achieve the ultimate aims of medicine: the aims of preserving life and of restoring health in the diseased or health-impaired human person. But, paradoxically, at the same time the new techniques and knowledge have come to be developed and used as direct threats to life and health. Current advances in scientific techniques are being absorbed from biology into human

19

medicine, and some of them have put in jeopardy the genuine ends of medicine – healing and caring – which give it its ultimate sense. The ancient Hippocratic principles encapsulated in the command 'Do not harm', which establish the basis for medical ethics, appear to be no longer absolute imperatives for medical practice.

The pressure in many countries on the medical profession to staff a State abortion service illustrates this point, as does the pressure on medical practitioners to comply with demands for the administration of contraceptive drugs even to the under-16s. For the suppression of ovulation by quantities of hormonal steroids is a very serious jolt to the workings of the body, involving as it does the disruption of the entire endocrine system. Long periods of such induced temporary sterility by steroids are now known to be connected with severe organic diseases such as cervical cancer, breast cancer, depression, immunological deficiencies, etc.[4] It is hard to see how the inducement of temporary sterility by drugs (affecting around 80 million women throughout the world), or the surgical inducement of permanent sterility, could ever be represented as an integral part of medical dedication to healing. They are more truly described as scientific possibilities, put in the hands of the medical profession whose consciences must be the final arbiters of what real healing is. For medicine is not at all the servant of scientific enterprise, not at all tied to doing what is scientifically possible. In view of these facts the following question is of the utmost importance for every medical practitioner: Is the Hippocratic ethic and tradition a matter of conscience for me? Each one of us needs to answer the question.

II. The new IVF technology: a brief history

6. Let me focus in particular on the recent development of the medico-scientific technique of human *in vitro* fertilisation (IVF). I shall begin with a brief consideration of the history of its development.

Although human IVF was first reported in the 1940s, by J. Rock and M. F. Menkin,[5] the history of the technique, as we have it today, may be considered to have had three related periods of development which began in the late 1950s.

(a) The first decade in the history of IVF dates from the late 1950s until 1968. It is a period of intense scientific research and study on the process of mammalian egg maturation, part of which was achieved by the method of *in vitro* maturation of the eggs of various animals as well as the human ovum.[6] Significant discoveries in this field were attained by Dr R. G. Edwards, who in 1965 reported the identification of the first meiotic division of the human egg[7] establishing that the process of egg maturation had begun. During this decade, *in vitro* methods were in the hands of research scientists, and were employed as part of a scientific enterprise. By 1966, Dr Edwards had written: 'Much of the fundamental work on oocyte maturation and some occasional examples of the fertilisation of these oocytes *in vitro* had been achieved ... I still recall working then with Dr Howard Jones in Baltimore, operating on a rhesus monkey to place human spermatozoa and mature human oocytes in the oviduct, in an attempt to obtain fertilisation.'[8]

(b) In the second decade of its history, from 1968 to 1978, IVF became a collaborative endeavour between scientists and clinicians. In 1968 the first medico-scientific research team was established by Dr Edwards (who is a physiologist), Dr Jean Purdy, his colleague at Cambridge, and Dr Patrick Steptoe, then a consultant at Oldham General Hospital. The team expressed the aim of its work as being 'To attempt [human] fertilisation *in vitro* and the culture of embryos in order to alleviate some forms of infertility, and to study the origin of inherited defects'.[9] In this ten-year period all the steps which were fundamental to the implementation of human IVF were successfully taken. They included the basic understanding and control of:
(i) the maturation of the human egg, follicle growth and the process of ovulation;
(ii) the fertilising capacitation of sperm;
(iii) the aspiration of the pre-ovulatory egg from its follicle;
(iv) fertilisation *in vitro*;
(v) the replacement of the embryo in the womb;

(vi) the implantation of the embryo in the womb and the continuation of pregnancy.

The mastering of these steps made possible the birth of the first baby conceived *in vitro*, Louise Brown, in July 1978.

(c) Between July 1978 and 1988, the third decade in the history of IVF, three major developments occurred: the opening of the Bourn Hall Clinic in Cambridgeshire by Dr Edwards and Dr Steptoe in October 1980; the emergence of a great number of centres all over the industrialised world where human IVF is practised; and the establishment of the procedure of multiple ovulation for the human female undergoing an IVF programme, together with the allied freeze-thaw procedure for human embryos, permitting their storage and also making possible large-scale experimentation upon them.

7. The achievements at Bourn Hall, when compared with those of all the other centres taken together, are quite remarkable. An example may illustrate this point. At Bourn Hall, from October 1980 to April 1983, embryos conceived *in vitro* were transferred to 1,200 women; as a result, 139 babies were born (67 boys and 73 girls).[10] By April 1983 there were, in the different parts of the industrialised world, about 250 babies who had been conceived *in vitro* and born (a year later, about 700 children were said to have been born by this method). So more than half of them in that early period were conceived and born at Bourn Hall in roughly 18 months.

Taking into consideration the thousands of embryos which, over the years, have been conceived *in vitro*, the thousands which, out of all these, have been transferred to their mothers and not destroyed in one way or another in the process of experimentation, and the number of embryos that have in fact implanted, developed to full term and been born, it is fair to draw the following conclusions. First, the IVF method, considered as a means to alleviate infertility, has noticeable limitations: if we are to rely on Bourn Hall figures – 1,200 women received embryos and 139 babies were born – the success rate was roughly 11 per cent, and it continues to be the same. Secondly, the method has involved, and continues to involve, the inevitable loss of thousands of embryos which are either directly used and destroyed in the process or which die because

22

of the process. Thirdly, the method does not, then, compare for efficiency with the natural method of conception and continuation of pregnancy, in which nature economically provides (except on rare occasions) just one egg for fertilisation: this comparative inefficiency has, in fact, been conceded recently by one practitioner of IVF.[11] It is common procedure at present in all teams working on IVF to replace in the womb more than one embryo – from two to five, or even more. This procedure greatly increases the chances of implantation of at least one of the embryos. But the reasons why this is the case are far from clear.[12]

8. It is said that the innumerable benefits to be derived from the study of human embryos and human gametes will be directly concerned with areas such as human conception and organogenesis, cancer, genetic defects, transplants, etc. It is claimed that the studies will make possible, for example, immunological contraception, abortion during the first month of pregnancy, selection of the sex of our future offspring, early diagnosis of genetic abnormalities and the use of embryonic tissue as well as of whole organs for transplantation; they will open up the way to inter-species breeding and gestation, and guide artificial manipulations in the early embryo so as to bring about cloning, artificial twinning, chimerism, etc. Yet the fact that all these alleged benefits are to be attained by experimenting on human embryos has been criticised by scientists themselves, and from a scientific point of view.[13] They have claimed that the benefits sought can be attained without the need to experiment directly on embryos at all. A thorough statement from expert geneticists would help enormously to clarify this important issue.

9. Because the practice of IVF has spread so rapidly over the industrialised world, numerous medical bodies have advanced ethical guidelines in this new field. The ethical and legal debate has become a matter of public concern. The rapid growth of deleterious practices, including destructive experimentation on human beings, is such that many governments of East and West have already legislated in these matters, or are about to do so.[14]

The main trends of the medico-ethical debate in Britain may be gathered from the guidelines issued by four British medical bodies: the Medical Research Council, the British Medical Association, the Ethics Committee of the Royal College of Obstetricians and Gynaecologists, and the Royal Society of Medicine. The main recommendations made by all these bodies are well represented in a document produced in June 1983 by the Standing Committee of the Joint European Medical Research Councils. The main points of the recommendations of the European body are as follows:

1. '. . . research on the process and pre-implantation products of *in vitro* fertilisation between gametes . . . can be supported.'
2. 'When human ova have been obtained and fertilised *in vitro* for a therapeutic purpose, and are no longer required for that purpose it would be acceptable to use them for . . . research.'
3. 'The fertilisation of ova in the laboratory [for purposes of research] is acceptable provided there is no intent to transfer the embryo . . .'
4. 'Studies on interspecies interaction involving human gametes are valuable . . . The product should not be allowed to develop beyond the early cleavage stages.' (*The Lancet*, 19 November, 1983, p. 1187.)

These recommendations have been accepted by the Medical Research Councils, or similar organisations, of Austria, Belgium, Denmark, Finland, France, the Federal Republic of Germany, Italy, the Netherlands, Portugal, Spain, Sweden, Switzerland and the United Kingdom. Ireland expressed strong reservations concerning recommendations 1 and 3. Norway proposed its own recommendations with more limitations.

10. It is crucially important to realise that the aim of scientists, medical practitioners and those others involved in the technique of IVF is, and always has been, the attainment of higher rates of human pregnancy (or the alleviation of infertility) as well as progress in scientific and medical knowledge. *Their primary aim has never been, and is not in current practice, to provide an opportunity for each generated embryo, that is, for each newly-conceived human being, to continue to live and follow its normal course of development.* It is in the actual *aim* with which

24

the technique started and continues to be practised that its basic moral deficiency lies. One of the *in vitro* pioneers has written: 'Embryos were grown during the early investigations without any intention of replacing them in the uterus, so that a minimum standard of success compatible with the introduction of a clinical programme to cure infertility could be attained.'[15] Likewise, the recommendations contained in the guidelines mentioned above do not have as their primary aim that of giving each generated embryo the opportunity to live and develop normally.

11. It is clear that there are two fundamental and related assumptions underlying the current ethical guidelines and practice of IVF. The first assumption is that *the early embryo does not enjoy full human status*; the second assumption, related to the first, is that *the value and interests of science and society override the value and interests of the newly-conceived human being*. The ground on which these assumptions rest constitutes the central problem of the present medico–ethical debate, a problem on which there is a great need for a conscientious position which is scientifically informed and fully developed with moral, philosophical and theological insight.

III. The Hippocratic perspective and the human conceptus

12. A concerted effort is being made to undermine the traditional moral positions of Hippocratic medicine, and to argue that science gives us no grounds for thinking that an embryo is anything more than a collection of cells with the potential to become human. It is alleged that we cannot reasonably believe, on the basis of biological facts about the nature of the human embryo, that the latter is a human person in embryonic form, and that there is no other way in which we could come to know that that is really the case. The presupposition here is that scientific knowledge is the only human knowledge which has the characteristic of certainty. There is no doubt that the present situation with reference to medical problems of life manifests a tension, and at times an open confrontation, between morals, philosophy and science.

25

The Declaration of Geneva, which dates back to 1948 and which is a contemporary version of the Hippocratic oath, demands of doctors the following commitment: 'I will maintain the utmost respect for human life from the time of conception'. In October 1983 the Assembly of the World Medical Association changed the Declaration, which now reads: 'I will maintain the utmost respect for human life from the time of commencement'. It is argued that '. . . precisely when and where life commences is left an open question', for, the argument continues, 'embryos are not only being aborted, they are also being grown *in vitro* . . .' (*The Lancet*, 10 December 1983, p. 1357). To leave open the *philosophical* question as to when the life of a human being begins is to leave open the *moral* question as to when he or she should begin to be respected. The decision to leave the question open is based, no doubt, on current practices; yet the type of theoretical justification given is precisely that in view of the biological facts, and in view of the new advances in scientific techniques, the question cannot be decided.

13. Let me dwell briefly on this presupposition and try to establish what, in general terms, we can expect of the biological (or, more generally, the scientific) facts. I distinguish, for the sake of convenience, between (a) what we may call 'the existential "that"', the *knowledge that* something or other is the case (for example, that something *is* or that something is a reality, that it exists as such-and-such a thing), and on the other hand (b) the scientific *knowledge how*, which refers to our ability to account for the structure and functioning of a living reality by the experimental methods of observing, measuring, dissecting, analysing, controlling, etc. It is by the use of these scientific methods that we seek to understand how things happen, how they are organised and work, how they are regulated and governed by laws. Let me illustrate this point. I know *that* I exist: my existence is a fact in the sense that it is something real. I also know that I have not always existed as a human being; I know that I must have had a beginning, which I do not recall; I know that I developed as a child, reached adulthood, that I am getting no younger and that I shall eventually die. I am absolutely certain *that* this is the case. Yet

26

I do not know *how* I, who am a person, full of spirit, understanding, self-direction, wondering about eternity and looking forward to it, could ever have come into existence with the fusion of an egg and a sperm. It is a mystery to me how I, as a person, could ever have come into existence as a tiny cell in a minute form. And what is more, I do not expect scientists ever to be able to tell me *how* this happens. I know *that* I remain the same person, even if most of the cells of my body change every six years or so. I also know that all these biological processes take care of themselves, and my conscious contribution to them is to eat, rest, move and not to worry too much. But *how* I remain the same person while my cells change is something which biologists will never tell me. Scientists cannot tell me how it happens that I am a person *and* a living organism all in one. They will, indeed, tell me something of how my organism works, but nothing about my being both a person and an organism. Biology has to take that reality for granted; it has no means of investigating it.

14. The point I want to make with these remarks is that what a human being really is, what his nature and identity really are, is no less of a mystery in the adult stages than in the embryonic or unborn stages of life. If you cut me open, or split me up, or flatten me down, you will always find a mass of organs constituted by cells, all with their chromosomes and my person-specific genes and DNA. If you flatten a human embryo you will ultimately see – as in my own case – cells and chromosomes and genes and DNA. Thus, from a biological point of view, the mystery about a tiny embryo being a person is no different from, or greater than, the mystery of your organism and mine being persons. Microscopes do not reveal personal identities; yet the reality of one's personal identity cannot be denied. In cutting me up, or looking with a microscope into the different tissues of my body, you will not find out more about the person that I am; nor will you find by this method whether the zygote or the embryo are persons or not. I am a cluster of cells as much as the embryo is. That is why, if I were a biologist or scientist, I would not be correct in maintaining that because I do not *know how* I am both a person and a living organism I do not *know that* I am one, or am uncertain whether

I am one, or am entitled to deny that I am one or to ignore this altogether. The fact that we do not know *how* a zygote or an embryo can be a person does not entitle us to claim *that* they are not. To think so is to blind ourselves to knowledge of realities which are not open to the scientific 'eye' but which are nevertheless clearly manifested to us. These realities make up the realm with which philosophy is concerned.

15. We know that at fertilisation the new individual, the embryo, becomes a distinct entity, containing *actually present* (and not merely potentially) that power within itself which will come in adulthood to full exercise and lead to full personal manifestation. We know that while the organism develops, the individual remains all the time the *same individual*. What anything can become is a possibility based on what that thing is. Thus the kind of life that a human embryo has, because of the dynamisms and capacities that it possesses *now*, is personal life, that is, the life of a personal being or a personal subject. The human embryo is an embryonic human person. Biological and philosophical knowledge and reflection complement each other. On the basis of that knowledge and reflection we have weighty evidence for maintaining this truth – that as members of the human species, as human persons, we came into being at conception – rather than its opposite. This evidence also tells us that the norm in nature is that each one of us has one unique genetic constitution, that is, that each person has genes which are person-specific. Also, each person is an individual organism, remaining the same from the time of his early zygotic form until the present stage of adulthood and eventually until death. Each one of us is an individual person, endowed with an eternal destiny. These three aspects of our individuality are unified in the one being that each of us is.

16. The idea that from conception the human individual should be respected has been expressed in a fundamental principle which has traditionally been called 'the principle of the sanctity of life', or (borrowing words from the Hippocratic Oath) as 'the principle of utmost respect for human life from the moment of conception'. Classic histories of medicine, such as that of H. Garrison, indicate that the medical

profession in the West has always been guided and inspired by this ideal of the Hippocratic tradition. There is no doubt that the wisdom and sensitivity expressed in the oath has been proved by the test of time. To change the spirit of the oath would be to change the *aims* of medicine – and not for the better – for it would change the principles on which the practice is based and which constitute medicine as a healing profession.

IV. Can there be a 'simple case' of IVF?

17. Let me draw your attention to an important question which illustrates the need for being well informed if one is to make conscientious evaluations and decisions. The question may be put thus: Can one say conscientiously that as regards *in vitro* conception there is at least one case in which this mode of conception is morally permissible? The most common answer to this question is in the affirmative. I want to elucidate and examine that answer.

A number of submissions made to the Warnock Committee expressed total acceptance of the principle of respect for the sacredness of every human life from its beginning at conception.[16] This is the most fundamental moral principle which underlies the recommendations contained in these submissions concerning current practices and future possibilities of human *in vitro* fertilisation, and it is based on the recognition that the highest value to be respected in our moral world is the individual human person. The paramount value of 'human life' – as we abstractly put it – means, in the concrete, the paramount value of every individual human being from conception to death. It is notable that these submissions, even though committed to respect for the sacredness of life, do not express any moral objection, on the basis of this commitment, to what is commonly called the 'simple case' or the 'straight case' in IVF. This is the case in which a married couple who are committed to the principle of respect for life from its beginning at conception seek the alleviation of their infertility by means of IVF. In this case the couple would request that one ovum be taken from the wife, that it be fertilised *in vitro* with the husband's sperm, and that, at the most appropriate

29

moment of its early development, the newly-conceived human being be transferred to his mother's womb. This 'simple case' was the one which applied in the conception of Louise Brown, the first test-tube baby, which Dr R. G. Edwards once described in the following terms: 'It was wonderful to collect the single egg, fertilise it *in vitro*, and watch it grow to an 8-cell embryo, when it was replaced in its mother.'[17]

18. At the present time, the 'simple case' in IVF is the one endorsed and recommended by a great number of those who do not want to abandon the principle of respect for every human life. It is considered that there is nothing seriously morally wrong with the 'simple case' of conception *in vitro*: the sanctity of life is preserved, family life, marital fidelity and marital union are not broken but enhanced. Therefore, it is thought, the 'simple case' may be permitted or recommended. Is this really so? In what follows I shall offer an answer to this question solely in the light of the requirements deriving from commitment to the principle of respect for the sacredness of life. The issues to be discussed are related (i) to the technical procedures themselves, and (ii) to the purposes and actions of the clinical team, that is, doctors, scientists, technicians and others.

19. For the lay person, *in vitro* conception is a simple idea: an ovum is taken from the woman's ovary, fertilised in a glass dish with the husband's sperm, and then the newly-conceived human being is transferred to his mother's womb. Yet anyone at all familiar with the actual technical process which achieves this form of conception is aware of the extraordinary complexities which are actually involved in the procedure. There are countless variables, connected with the natural biological mechanisms of fertility and generation, that need to be controlled, some of which, although basic, are not even known as yet – for example, some crucial factors influencing implantation. The present low success rate in achieving pregnancies by the IVF method is due to these still-unknown mechanisms and uncontrolled variables, and to the complexity of the process which involves great stress for the patient,

constant monitoring, the use of drugs and a surgical operation with total anaesthesia. Because of the very technical nature of the method, the gametes, that is, the sperm and the egg, as well as the embryonic human being, have to be handled with instruments and machines and exposed to artificial environments, e.g., differences in light and temperature, in time processes, in culture medium, and so on. In practice all this carries with it, for the embryonic human being, either the risk of death, that is, of being killed during the process (for many more embryos die in the process than survive it), or the risk of serious and irreparable harm, that is, of being seriously damaged in the process or by the process (for many embryos begin to develop abnormally). These risks can never, in principle, be excluded.

20. Let me focus now on the purposes and means adopted so far by clinicians and scientists who have achieved *in vitro* conception in the so-called 'simple case'. It was mentioned above that the pioneers of the IVF method required approximately 20 years of study and experiment to attain the birth of the first test-tube baby in 1978. During that time human embryos were used and experimented upon without there being any intention of replacing them in the uterus. At present doctors and scientists maintain that in order to improve IVF methods and particularly to achieve higher rates of pregnancy, extra embryonic human beings must be brought into existence to be used and experimented upon. This is so because the clinical aim of the method is successful pregnancy, even if in the process newly-conceived human beings are to be harmed or have to be sacrificed. What matters is the end-result and the improvement of the method. Science and 'progress' come first; the dignity of the individual human being is subservient to them. It is important to note that there is no team working in IVF which openly adheres to the principle of respect for every human being. Their aims are successful pregnancies and the progress of science; newly-conceived human beings are therefore regarded as expendable for these purposes.

21. *The intrinsic nature of the technique.* There is no way in which scientists and doctors can guarantee that death or serious and irreparable damage will not be caused to the newly-conceived

31

human being, in the process or by the process of conception outside the womb *in vitro*. This is a fact intrinsic to the nature of the technique. Doctors now say that the degree of abnormality in children born through the IVF technique is not greater than in those born by natural conception. Sadly, they are not fully honest: they do not tell us the number of abnormal embryos they have destroyed and continue to destroy prior to transfer to the womb. Their comments, therefore, apply only to embryos that have been actually inplanted. For it is their *mandatory* policy that all embryos seen, or suspected, to be developing abnormally are not implanted but rather discarded (and therefore killed) – perhaps after having been experimented upon.[18] Moreover, the risk of serious damage to the child-to-be, inherent in the technique even if it were perfected, is acknowleged by medical guidelines such as those of the (British) Royal College of Obstetricians and Gynaecologists: 'the possibility that a child born with an abnormality might in due course be able to sue its parents and the doctors cannot be ruled out'.[19] In fact, as we all know, the principle 'Defectives should not be born' is part of an ethos, currently widespread, which does not accord respect to the intrinsic value of every human being. That is why a current back-up method for abnormal embryos is test-tube abortion, or, if need be, later abortion.

22. In the light of these facts, what ethical judgement should we pass upon the 'simple case' in IVF? If a couple who are seeking a successful pregnancy share the doctor's aim and attitudes as I have described them above, they have already abandoned the moral commitment of respect for every human being. In these circumstances, and given the attitude to the individual human being which is involved, it does not make much sense to talk in all earnestness about the 'simple case'. Furthermore, if a couple wish that only one ovum be taken from the wife, be fertilised *in vitro* with the husband's sperm, and then be transferred to the mother's womb, they would have to look for a team willing to conform to these requirements; and the fact is that there does not seem to be such a team at present. The aim of existing clinical teams is to achieve a pregnancy with the most economical and the least

troublesome means, even if countless newly-conceived human beings have to be harmed, to die, or to be disposed of in the process. To achieve that aim, the teams employ the practice of induced superovulation. In some clinics as many as 15 ova have been taken from a woman's ovary in one single monthly cycle, after she has been given a strong dose of hormones to induce the ripening of so many ova. All these ova are then fertilised, some embryos are implanted, and others are used in a variety of ways. Just the act of giving a strong dose of hormones to induce superovulation could have harmful effects on the eggs, and subsequently on the embryos, some of which could develop abnormally and therefore be killed. Further, when three or more embryos are transferred to the womb it is done in the knowledge (and so with the will) that one or two embryos may serve simply to assist the other(s) to survive. Hence some human beings are clearly being used as a mere means to the survival of others; indeed they are not cared for and respected for their own intrinsic value. Obstetricians clearly believe that if multiple pregnancies become the normal procedure as a result of *in vitro* conception, they will in fact constitute a serious risk for mother and children. In fact this has come to be the case.

23. Let us, however, assume that there is a clinical team willing to comply with the desires of those who wish only one egg to be taken from the wife, fertilised *in vitro* and then implanted. A crucial question of moral significance for the couple and the team arises even in this case. What if the embryo – the newly-conceived human being – is seen to be developing abnormally? What are the possible choices? Would replacement of the embryo in the mother's womb be the course to take if it were known that the child conceived would develop with abnormalities? Or would the embryo then be discarded and destroyed? Even if the parents wanted the abnormally-developing embryo to be replaced in the mother's womb, the clinical team would not comply with the parents' request. The possible medical, legal and social consequences of doing so would be regarded as intolerable. As already noted, it is now a matter of course for clinical teams to discard embryos which are developing abnormally. The parents' wishes are not

decisive here, for doctors 'are taking part in the formation of the embryo itself' – as the report of the Royal College of Obstetricians and Gynaecologists states (section 6.1) – and therefore 'that role brings a special sense of responsibility for the welfare of the child thus conceived'.

24. It is clear, then, that both doctors and parents, by embarking on a process of IVF conception which may cause irreparable harm to a child thus conceived, are adopting two kinds of related choices. First, they accept, and therefore choose, that if the newly-conceived embryo is defective it is to be discarded and killed. Secondly, they accept, and so choose, to give life to a child in conditions which involve serious risk of death or of irreparable damage to the child. Neither of the two choices is morally justifiable. It is clear that neither the clinical team nor the parents intentionally act (in the ideal case) so as to generate an abnormal embryo, or in order to place it in a situation in which it will be killed by the process. Rather, the high risks of causing harm or death are foreseeable consequences of IVF in the 'simple case'. Nonetheless, they are foreseeable consequences of an extremely grave kind, and only the gravest of reasons would justify one in freely bringing those consequences about. What reason could justify one in voluntarily causing serious harm or death to the newly-conceived human being, brought about in the process of his or her own generation? Can the existence, bodily integrity and well-being of the child be subservient to the desires of his or her progenitors?

25. Some would maintain that in nature the complexity and vulnerability of the process of conception is such that many human embryos in fact die, particularly those suffering from abnormalities. Hence, it is argued, we are entitled to use IVF as a mode of conception, in which the abnormal embryos can be 'allowed to die', just as they may die in the natural process. This argument ignores two important points. First, in the natural process of generation the child conceived with abnormalities may or may not abort and die. Second, it must be remembered that physical nature is not a moral agent, a person who is capable of making decisions on moral grounds, but that we are such agents. What we choose to do is in our control and

34

hence is our responsibility. The results of natural physical processes, which are not under our voluntary control, are not our responsibility. We are moral beings; physical nature is not. There really cannot be a 'simple case' of *in vitro* fertilisation. IVF is not a morally permissible mode of generation for those who are committed to cherishing and caring for every individual human being from conception to death; IVF is not a course open to those who want to give life and love to a child just for his own sake, as is appropriate and right in the case of a human person.

V. Conclusion: three general moral principles

26. By way of conclusion let me state some of the general principles of that basic Hippocratic ethic which is orientated to our genuine well-being.

(i) The foundation of any ethic, its ultimate source and arbiter, resides in *the primacy of the individual conscience*. The conscientious human person, always seeking what is true and what is good and acting accordingly, is the only route for reaching moral truth, that is, recognition of what is of genuine value.

(ii) A truly conscientious person recognises that the highest value to be respected in our human moral world – upon which any other value itself depends – is the individual human being. The Hippocratic tradition, as it is enshrined in modern times in the Declaration of Helsinki, categorically defends this idea of the paramount value of the individual human person. It stated that the interests of the individual subject cannot be overridden by the interests of science or society.

(iii) The Hippocratic outlook established the beginning of European medical ethics with its basic principle: 'Do not harm'. Many current medical practices are obvious causes of direct harm to human beings, even to the extent of direct killing. It is the duty of every individual clinician not to engage in any activity that by harming others ultimately jeopardises his own moral integrity. It is also his conscientious responsibility to safeguard the genuine ends of the medical profession, which make it the healing profession.

If the Hippocratic ethic is still alive it is because conscientious healers have lived by its truth and goodness for more than 2,000 years. May it continue to be so.

2

IVF: Ethical issues and social implications

I. Setting the scene: central questions and problems

1. One of the most important decisions that our government will have to make in the near future is concerned with the legal status of the human embryo.[1] The government's future decision, as well as the resolution of the basic social and ethical issues raised by the practice of human fertilisation *in vitro* (IVF), will depend, if it is reasonably and fairly made, on the moral status of the human embryo. That is to say, everything will turn on the answer we give to this question: What kind of respect is due to the human embryo? Is the human embryo to be protected as a human being or should it be regarded as a kind of property? Legal and public policy issues are not independent of moral evaluations or of facts: they ultimately rest upon them.

2. The recognition of facts and the moral evaluations we make in the course of answering this question concerning the status of the embryo will be of enormous significance, not only for the life of this nation but also for the world at large. The human family is, at this stage in history, already bound and knitted together as a whole. Not only economic and nuclear policies, but also policies regarding health and biomedical research adopted by countries with extensive technical and industrial resources, like this one, will eventually affect millions of human beings, for good or ill. Our responsibilities for our fellow human beings are no longer national, they are now of world-wide character, affecting the human family as a

whole. Every personal and social decision sets a standard. By such decisions we construct the moral climate of our world. Britain has been a pioneer in the development of IVF techniques; the moral and legal stand which this country now takes concerning the aims and procedures of this technique will inevitably be significant for the rest of the world as well. Britain cannot ignore this responsibility or be blind to it.

3. Let me introduce what seem to me to be the three most fundamental ethical issues related to the aims and procedures of IVF programmes, namely the questions of (a) the 'spare' embryos in the IVF and embryo replacement (ER) programme; (b) the experimental character of this programme; and (c) the practice, which it involves, of experimenting directly on human embryos, for scientific purposes. We shall consider later some of the social implications of these issues. I shall begin by referring briefly to Dr R. G. Edwards's own formulation of the problems, and to his ethical opinions – not only because Dr Edwards has from the beginning presented these opinions openly for discussion but also because they have had considerable influence on those who have formulated IVF guidelines at national and international levels.[2]

4. In 1969, Dr R. G. Edwards identified some of the medical and scientific possibilities opened up by study of and experimental research upon human embryos, activities in which he and others were then beginning to engage.[3] These possibilities were: the alleviation of human infertility; the development of new means of contraception (including even the 'immunisation' of people against fertilisation or implantation[4]); alleviation of genetic diseases and deformities and of other forms of disease; and further advances in the knowledge of human reproduction and of embryology in general.

(a) *The question of 'spare' embryos.* For Dr Edwards the basic ethical question in connection with the therapeutic aim of IVF and embryo replacement to alleviate human infertility was seen as early as 1969 in these terms: 'We would have to take several eggs from the mother, and transfer only one or two back into her. The remainder would be thrown away. Is it acceptable to discard the excess embryos?'[5] It is important to

37

note that this question was considered then, and is still considered now, as a fundamental *ethical* question. This is so because we are implicitly recognising that the embryo we are dealing with is human in a particular way, that is, that it is not mere 'human tissue', 'a cluster of cells' or 'a speck of matter'. If that were all the human embryo was, the question would be of little interest: a mere speck of human tissue of no relevance to the identity of the individual human being could not raise fundamental ethical and legal questions.

At present a number of arguments are advanced for the view that the practice of discarding embryos, or, alternatively, the practice of freezing them, is ethically acceptable; but perhaps at the root of all attempted justifications lies the one that Dr Edwards gave in 1969: '. . . by throwing the excess embryos away, we are doing no more than any couple using the intrauterine device for contraception . . . In a society which sanctions the abortion of a fully-formed fetus, the discarding of such a minute, undifferentiated embryo should be acceptable to most people.'[6] Indeed this is the case. But we know that acceptability by most people does not make a practice morally right, that counting heads is not a proper way to determine what is good or evil.[7] On the other hand we also know that the fact that a practice is socially accepted does indeed tend to influence people's moral attitudes, even if the change is not morally for the better. We are all exposed and vulnerable in this respect.

(b) *The experimental character of IVF and embryo replacement.* This question has not been raised as a specifically ethical question by those directly involved in the IVF programmes, but it has been raised by others,[8] both during the early stages of its development and at present. It is true that the current situation as regards IVF differs greatly from the early one in its achievements, which have been attained after 'the lonely and frustrating pathway that ultimately led to the joy of the birth of Louise Brown',[9] to use Dr Edwards's own words. Yet the ethical issues remain with us, and some more acutely so because of the advances. Despite the advances, many scientific uncertainties remain,[10] showing that this form of human generation entails serious risks, particularly for the child-to-be. Dr Edwards holds, with other researchers, that because the 'evidence of the liveborn children confirms observations in animals [which indicate] that the culture of pre-implantation embryos *in vitro* is safe and imposes no extra risks on the child . . ., the procedure could be introduced into clinical medicine with very few reservations, especially with the back-up screening provided by ultrasonic scans, amniocentesis and other tests in later pregnancy.'[11] It is revealing that despite Dr Edwards's optimism, certain reservations about possible risks involved in the IVF procedure are still present, the more so since the practice of freezing the spare embryos is now used.[12] The 'back-up' procedures must be viewed in the light of their ultimate aims. It must also be noted that it is normal practice in IVF-ER programmes not to implant the newly-fertilised embryo if it is developing abnormally.[13] In view of this fact alone the moral acceptability of any IVF therapeutic programme may be questioned.

(c) *Experimenting with human embryos and the study of embryology.* In 1981 the first internationally-attended meeting at Bourn Hall in Cambridge took place. It gathered authorities on IVF from this country, Switzerland, West Germany, Sweden, Australia, the United States, France and Austria.[14] It was there that the real possibility was acknowledged of growing embryos *in vitro* up to the stage where the early beginnings of organic differentiation occur: 'analyses on differentiation and early organogenesis in the human embryo are now feasible'.[15] Dr Edwards also pointed out that 'Better methods may be devised for culturing embryos *in vitro*, and the nature of normal and abnormal growth could be analysed. Methods might be introduced to use embryonic tissues for the cellular repair of damaged tissues in adults, especially for organs without renewal of stem cells.'[16] 'Will these methods and aims be ethically acceptable?', Dr Edwards asks. The answer he gives now is the same as the one he gave in 1969, and the justification which he now provides for this stance is also the same as it was then: 'The ethical issues involved in establishing and studying early embryos *in vitro* should be acceptable in view of the potential advantages of this work. These issues seem to be minor in relation to other ethical dilemmas involving embryos and fetuses, e.g. the accepted and widespread use of I.U.D.s and abortion for family limitation.'[17] The central ethical question raised by the scientific impetus behind the IVF programme was put by Dr Edwards to his colleagues at the Bourn Hall symposium in these terms: 'We have to make a decision as to whether human embryology should be pursued for its own sake.'[18]

5. Because the decisions to be taken are legal, moral and social in character, they affect us all. There is a great need for co-operative dialogue, weighty and truthful consideration of the facts and unswerving personal commitment to moral integrity – even though these are rare virtues – at a time when such crucial decisions are to be made. What routes may we take in order to come to such decisions? How are the aims and procedures, the means and ends, of IVF and of the study of embryology, to be assessed? We seem forced here to recognise and to consider certain truths related to two basic dimensions of our mode of being: truths of a moral order and truths of a biological order. In the light of these truths, personal moral decisions will have to be made which will determine our standpoint in respect of legislation and of practices in our present and future social lives. Obviously, the kind of decisions which each of us will make is something which depends on the attitudes which we freely adopt and which are embedded in our modes of thinking and living which enable us to recognise (or which hinder us from recognising) what is true.

II. Fundamental truths to be recognised: of moral order, of biological order

6. *Truths of moral order.* Central to our moral decisions and judgements is our basic moral vision, that is, the moral perspective by means of which we judge our own actions and the actions of other people to be right or wrong. Part of this moral vision is our attitude towards human life, that is, the way we regard and value each and every one of our fellow human beings. Our commitment to 'humanity', to its overall good and progress, necessarily takes the concrete form of a commitment to, or, alternatively, of a disregard for, this or that individual human being. Thus our personal moral attitude

40

could be summed up as amounting to 'what we would be prepared to do, or do in fact do, to any individual human being, including ourselves'.

7. A basic truth concerning our moral dealings with our fellow human beings is that they are not things that can be bought and sold, traded off, disposed of, produced to specified requirements and rejected when those requirements are no longer met. The worth of the human being demands a kind of respect which is not due to things. To treat the human being as a thing is to adhere to the 'slavery ethic' which, as involving a total denial of any moral worth in the human individual, is unjust and therefore immoral. The recognition that the human being is not a thing is the recognition that he or she should be treated not as a thing but rather with a kind of respect which is appropriate to his or her being. This respect is a fundamental requirement of justice, in virtue of which no human being is to be used or exploited for any purpose whatsoever. It is a recognition that *every human being has at least the right not to be used merely as a means to the needs or interests of others and every innocent human being has at least the right not to be killed.*[19] 'Not to be used, not to be killed' is the ultimate moral ground where the roots of justice lie. Recognition of this basic right amounts to an ultimate moral obligation for those of us who *can* actually use or actually kill others.

8. The inviolability of the individual human being has been part of the moral vision that the medical profession in its attempt to serve life has expressed in its codes of practice. The Hippocratic Code sets the principle *primum non nocere* right at 'the beginning of medical ethics'.[20] The code says: 'I will keep the sick from harm and injustice'. Not to harm, not to commit injustice: in order to follow this injunction one must, at the very least, refuse to use or damage anyone in the most radical way, that is, by destroying or killing him or her.

9. The World Medical Association, in its *Declaration of Helsinki* (1964; revised 1975), which is concerned with recommendations to doctors in biomedical research involving human subjects, adopts the same attitude towards respect for the life

of the individual human being. The Declaration states that 'Concern for the interests of the subject must always prevail over the interest of science and society'.[21] The final words of the Declaration are: 'In research on man, the interest of science and society should never take precedence over considerations related to the well-being of the subject'.[22]

10. It is not only that the historical social struggle for the abolition of slavery and racialism, our declarations and bills of rights, the law and medical codes of practice bear witness to the paramount value of the individual human being; in fact, the recognition of this value, and the moral demand to act in accordance with it, constitutes a cornerstone or first principle of traditional moral philosophies. As Kant said, we must never treat a human being as a mere means but always as an end.

11. The moral thinking of the Jewish-Christian tradition has incorporated this same vision and continues to do so: 'Love thy neighbour' is a basic commandment. By 'neighbour' is understood any human being; by 'love', the measure of respect, care and responsibility for another which not only rules out any act of injustice against him, but is even capable of generating the commitment to give one's own life for him.

12. It must be recalled, however, that for the utilitarian tradition in philosophy (much adopted in this country, in principle and in practice), respect for the individual human being is not the paramount moral value; the paramount moral value is rather 'the greatest good of the greatest number'. On this view there will be circumstances in which the lives of individual human beings may be regarded as instrumental, and so as expendable, for the sake of that 'greater good'. Ultimately, in utilitarianism, all values, including the lives of human beings, can be 'traded off'.[23] This is not so for the non-utilitarian outlook I have been presenting, and to which I adhere. Within this latter outlook any weighing and comparing of values occurs only as governed by the presupposition that respect for the inviolability of each individual human being is under no

circumstances to be 'traded off', that is, that the direct killing of an innocent human being is never justifiable.

13. *Truths of biological order.* The biological sciences can tell us today that a new human being, a new member of the human species, comes into existence at fertilisation. I take the following claims to be well and truly justified on the basis of the scientific evidence. The cell is at once the universal component of all living bodies and the factor that unites one generation to the next. The human body is constituted by two kinds of cells, the somatic and the generative. Those of the first kind contain 46 chromosomes, the number of chromosomes proper to the human species. The generative cells contain half that number, 23. The ovum and the sperm are cells of the latter kind and are capable of establishing the link between one human generation and the next. They are the cells which are active in bringing about human reproduction. When an ovum and a sperm unite and their pronuclei fuse, a new single cell comes into being, the most remarkable of all cells. Its coming into existence reveals both the baffling mystery and the comprehensibility of human life. Let me quote Francois Jacob's vision of this cell:

> The formation of a man from an egg is a marvel of exactitude and precision. How can millions and millions of cells emerge, in specialised lineages, in perfect order in time and space, from a single cell? This baffles the imagination. During embryonic development, the instructions contained in the chromosomes of the egg are gradually translated and executed, determining when and where the thousands of molecular species that constitute the body of an adult are to be formed. The whole plan of growth, the whole series of operations to be carried out, the order and the site of syntheses and their co-ordination are all written down in the nucleic-acid message. And in the execution of the plan, there are few failures: the accuracy of the system may be measured by the rarity of abortions and monsters.[24]

14. When we consider the differences and similarities between, on the one hand, the individual cells, ovum and sperm, and, on the other, the zygote which arises from their union, we find that some significant facts emerge. One is connected with the question: When does human life begin? A biologist has answered the question thus: 'Never. Life ends often, but it

never begins. It is just passed on from one cell to another. All biologists . . . are in agreement on that answer.'[25] Indeed, not only life but humanity is a continuum. For an ovum must be a living, mature human cell to be fertilised by a sperm, which must also be alive and human to bring about a new living human cell: the zygote. The specifically human character and life of the ovum and sperm have been received from other cells. Thus the question 'When does human life begin?' must strictly be answered: 'It does not begin, it is continuous, it is transmitted.'

It is important to note that life exists only in individuals of specific forms, that is, it exists and is communicated only in and through the individual organisms that constitute the members of this or that species. This is a fact. So a legitimate question arises: When does 'human life' become a human being? When does a new human organism, a new member of the species, come into existence? The biological sciences have answered this question in a definite way: at fertilisation, neither before nor after.[26] At fertilisation a new, unique, complete human organism begins to exist. It is human like all the other cells, but its humanity differs in kind from that of other cells. Biologists have put it this way:

A zygote is human because within its total DNA conformation are the DNA structures which determine, and are common to, the human species. It is a specific human being because the total DNA conformation of this individual is constant at all points of the organism's existence.[27]

15. So it is not true to say that 'Everything that can be said about the potential of the embryo can also be said of the potential of the egg and sperm'.[28] First, the genetic constitution of the zygote is not that of the egg and sperm. The 46 chromosomes in the zygote are a different kind of reality from the 23 in the sperm and the ovum considered together. Secondly, the zygote is from the beginning a genetically complete, organised, unique individual organism in the species. If it does not die and is not killed, it will develop into a man or a woman. This is not the destiny of ovum and sperm if they do not unite. Thirdly, the process of development and its finality is inbuilt in the power of the new organism itself;

this development of a human being may be described as 'a process of becoming the one he already is'.[29] That is why I can truly say that my life as an adult is continuous with my life as a child, and my life as a zygote. I am trillions of cells now, but once I began as a single cell, a zygote. Yet I have never been an unfertilised ovum, nor a sperm. The beginning of me must be traced back to fertilisation, when a particular sperm and ovum came together to cause a substantial change – the beginning of me. Thus the continuity between the adult bodily selves we are and the embryonic bodily selves we were is today a matter of established fact. The human being as a member of his species comes into existence at fertilisation and ceases to exist when he dies. This much biology can tell us.

16. According to Professor Peter Singer,

> When opponents of abortion say that the embryo is a living human being from conception onwards, all they can possibly mean is that the embryo is a living member of the species *homo sapiens*. This is all that can be established as a scientific fact. But is this also the sense in which every 'human being' has a right to life?[30]

Professor Singer answers the question in the negative: to be a human being does not amount to having a right to life – that is, to having an entitlement to human moral status. A similar line has been taken by the Medical Research Council, by the Ethical Committee of the Royal College of Obstetricians and Gynaecologists and by the British Medical Association in their guidelines concerning IVF, embryo replacement and embryo transfer. This moral option is characteristic of the utilitarian tradition. It is an option that carries with it other fundamental options: it is necessarily a commitment to the view that not all human beings are equal; that *humanity* is not the universal ground of our equal status; that there are some human beings whose humanity is rightly judged to be of a 'lesser kind', either because of their merely incipient organic development or because of some defective or damaged organic condition. The option is also a commitment to the view that these 'lesser human beings' can legitimately be used as instruments for the benefit and interests of others who are more adequately

45

endowed – either because they already have a central nervous system, or look human, or have already been born, or are adults who can reason and exercise autonomy. So the rights of the 'lesser' human beings will be subservient to the rights of the 'full' human beings. Thus (as the RCOG Report puts it, following the position taken by Dr Edwards) when we have a situation in which a living child requires a bone marrow transplant obtainable from an embryo, 'the rights of the 14-day embryo should be subservient to the interests of the living child' (Section 13.7). Here one would like to know, with Mr David Bolt of the BMA Council, just what there is that is so sacrosanct about the 14th day.[31] Naturally, the lesser human beings will legally become a sort of property and will be used and disposed of accordingly.

17. The option to disregard humanity as the basis of moral status amounts to a departure from the egalitarian ideal that has led us to the abolition of slavery and is leading us to the abolition of any kind of apartheid. It also signals a departure from 'the respect for life from the time of conception'[32] which is expected of clinicians and researchers in their tradition and their medical codes of practice. It is, moreover, a departure from the vision of the human individual which is inherent in our laws and in common morality: as an end in himself and not (as the utilitarian outlook views him) an instrument to be used to serve the interests of others. I cannot accept such a departure from common moral principles or the new moral vision that prompts it. The biological determination of the moment when a new human being comes into existence, and the moral vision recognising that a human being is not a piece of property and so is not to be used or exploited for any purpose whatever, provide us with firm grounds for including in the human family all human beings, from conception to death, as sharing the human moral status which entitles them to have their lives protected. The human embryo is indeed a member of the species, a human being. The respect owed to our embryonic selves, to the earliest stages of our lives, should not differ in kind from the respect owed to any member of the human family, for we all share the same human condition. This respect implies, at the very least, the right 'not to be used

as a mere means to the interests of others, and [the right] not to be killed'.[33]

III. Aims and means of IVF: what is permissible, what is desirable

18. The opening questions of my paper – What kind of respect is due to the human embryo? Is the human embryo to be protected as a human being or as a piece of property? – have been answered in this paper in the following way. The respect due to the human embryo does not differ in kind from the respect due to any other human being; the human embryo must be protected as a human being and not regarded as an object of use or as someone's property.

In the light of these answers, how are we to assess the aims of IVF programmes and the means which are taken to fulfil those aims?

(i) Embryology for its own sake?

19. Let me begin by considering the ethical question raised by Dr Edwards: Should human embryology be pursued for its own sake? An affirmative answer is at present defended on the basis of arguments such as the following. It is desirable to learn as much as possible about human reproduction, organogenesis and the function of genes; it is desirable to improve knowledge that will help to treat genetic and chromosomal abnormalities as well as infertility; it is desirable, therefore, that research be carried out on human embryos, because such knowledge is not obtainable in any other way.

Let us assume for the moment that these are all worthy aims and that lesser aims such as some that Professor William Walters and Professor Singer might entertain – concerning, for example, the development of animal-human hybrids who 'would be able to carry out unpleasant jobs and mundane tasks in the community, relieving man for more skilled occupations'[34] – are excluded.

These worthy aims are all to be carried out at the cost of the lives of human beings, even if they are lives in their early beginnings. The ends (on this view) justify the means; and the

47

principles that at present justify those means and aims will justify more radical ones. There is no reason why they could not be extended further, even if more human beings, at a more developed stage in their lives, are to be utilised. It is not surprising, then, that many scientific researchers take the attitude that there should be no restrictions on research at all.[35]

On moral grounds the question 'Embryology for its own sake?', understood as explained above, must be answered in the negative. Studying and experimenting on human embryos for scientific purposes is immoral. *For such experiments are never in the interest of the subject experimented upon*, who is harmed, used up and destroyed: he or she is always used radically as a means, as an object of use. Thus, practices such as embryo division, freezing of embryos, observing the development of human embryos and fetuses *in vitro*, the generation and growth of embryos *in vitro* for tissue culture and transplantation, genetic manipulation of embryos, and attempts to bring about cloning, ectogenesis (i.e., the continuing development of the fetus *in vitro*) and hybridisation (i.e., trans–species fertilisation) are all radical instrumentalisations of human beings. They are radically immoral.

(ii) Generation of 'spare embryos'?

20. Perhaps what we might all consider as acceptable in the IVF programmes is the therapeutic aim of alleviating the infertility of a married couple. Yet in order to achieve this admittedly good aim, unethical means must also be endorsed in practice, for there must be some use or disposal of 'spare' embryos. The spare embryos are usually obtained by the method of induced superovulation in the woman. The practice of inducing superovulation is justified on the following grounds: (i) it avoids subjecting the woman to the trauma and hazard of repeated laparoscopies for recovering ova (such a surgical operation requires total anaesthesia); (ii) superovulation facilitates the selection of embryos before implantation; (iii) it also increases the possibility of attaining the aim of the programme, that of achieving pregnancy, for if there is a miscarriage one of the spare embryos may then be implanted; (iv) if ova were always to be recovered only at the moment

that ovulation normally takes place in each woman's menstrual cycle, a heavy burden would be placed on the team of doctors who would have to be available at that particular time.[36]

It is indeed clear that the generation of spare embryos is the most economical procedure for attaining the general aim in view – the greatest possible chance of pregnancy with the minimum of effort, expense and trauma. Yet the well-being and existence of each individual human being thus generated is made secondary and instrumental to the general aim. Those embryonic human beings, if not required for the desired pregnancy, will be disposed of, used for experiments or frozen until a time comes when they will again be demanded for implantation, experimentation or disposal.

21. We noted earlier Dr Edwards's claim that the disposal or usage of embryos is justified since many other early human lives are destroyed for less worthy purposes by means of IUDs or in eugenic abortion (and those abortions carried out not to protect the life of the mother but for the sake of limiting the family or for the interest of society).[37] Naturally, this raises the question of whether the direct destruction of any human being, whether by IUD, abortion, disposal or experimentation, is justified. Dr Edwards seems to imply that a society which accepts eugenic abortion has no moral grounds for prohibiting experimentation on embryos. In my opinion he is right on this point. This whole question also shows how far and into what new fields the acceptance of abortion can reach.

22. A different type of justification at present being offered for the disposal of spare embryos is this: 'Knowing as we do that in the natural process large numbers of fertilised ova are lost before implantation, it is unreasonable to claim absolute inviolability for an organism with which nature itself is so prodigal.'[38] It is clear to us all, I think, that natural processes such as volcanic eruptions, floods, droughts and other kinds of natural disasters may destroy hundreds of human lives, as well as animal lives. These are natural processes as much as the processes whereby the loss of fertilised ova naturally occur. Can these natural processes really be taken as indicative of what we

are to do? Someone giving an affirmative answer to this question would have to ignore the fact that what we intend, decide and deliberately bring about are not natural processes – and that just because they are not natural processes, we are answerable for them. They cannot be measured against the natural results that nature brings about. We are moral beings; physical nature is not. The life of a human being, at whatever stage of its development, may come naturally to an end. No one is morally accountable for that. But if we voluntarily bring about the death of that individual, or bring him or her into existence with that ultimate intention, we are morally accountable for such an intention and such an action. What physical nature does is no ultimate moral standard or excuse for us. There is no moral justification for our directly killing human beings, using them as objects, instrumentalising them or exploiting them for any purpose whatever.

(iii) Grave risk of harm or death for those conceived by IVF?

23. What should we say of the *therapeutic* aim of IVF, its use for the purpose of alleviating infertility in a married couple when disposal or usage of spare embryos is not involved in the programme? What moral judgement should we make concerning this 'simple case' of IVF, as it has been called? Even in this case I find serious ethical objections to the programme, these objections centring on the possibly irreparable harm to the child-to-be. (See above, Chapter One, para. IV.) At present, it is claimed that children born following IVF do not suffer from congenital abnormalities to any greater extent than do children conceived in natural circumstances.[39] However, this fact does not resolve the important ethical issues which arise for those who want to follow the IVF programme and who are also committed to respecting human life from its very beginning. (For the numerical data indicating the rate of abnormality and death of embryos generated by IVF, see Chapter Seven below, para. 17.) The following situation provides an illustration of this. What would be the position of a couple who, following the IVF programme in order to overcome infertility, find that after fertilisation the

new embryo is developing abnormally? Would they choose to go ahead and replace the embryo in the womb for implantation, knowing that the child conceived would grow up with congenital abnormalities? Or would the embryo instead be destroyed? Doctors now follow the policy of not implanting embryos which are developing abnormally. The parents cannot have the last decision in this issue, for doctors are not merely enablers in the process of IVF, but, as the RCOG Report notes, 'They are taking part in the formation of the embryo itself. That role brings a special sense of responsibility for the welfare of the child thus conceived' (Section 6.1). Thus it is inherent in the nature of the IVF technique that irreparable damage to the embryo or the child-to-be cannot be excluded. This is clearly acknowledged by Dr Edwards when he mentions the back-up methods of monitoring abnormalities after IVF and implantation, as well as implicitly by the RCOG when it says that 'the possibility a child born with an abnormality might in due course be able to sue its parents and the doctors cannot be ruled out' (Section 10.7).

24. Are we morally justified in bringing about a process with such a risk of harm? My answer is in the negative and is shared by P. Ramsey[40] and L. Kass,[41] and by H. Teifel.[42] It is no excuse for us to say that abnormalities following IVF are similar to those following the natural process of conception. Again: nature takes care of itself, but we have to take care of *our* actions. A child brought into existence with an abnormality resulting from conception *in vitro*, where human responsibility and knowledge have directly intervened, cannot accept it in the same way as a child whose handicap results from a purely natural process. If the well-being of each individual child were always the crucial consideration, rather than the wishes of the parents, no-one would embark on such risky generation. An attitude of respect for the human being, not seeking to use him or her as a means for the interests of others in any circumstances, must lead us to hold that just as 'a malformed infant has the same rights as a normal infant',[43] so a mal-developing embryo should be afforded the same respect and protection as that which is due to a well-developing embryo. To embark on processes where both normal

51

embryos and defective embryos are generated and some must be discarded is immoral.

25. It seems clear that respect for and protection of the human embryo in accord with its human status can be guaranteed only in the natural process of procreation and not in the technical IVF mode of generation, because the mal-forming embryo will never have the chance of being treated with respect: it is bound to be killed; it will not be implanted. If it were to be implanted in the knowledge that it was abnormal, it would be found practically impossible to bear the moral and legal responsibilities involved.[44] In a natural process of pro-creation such an embryo might or might not abort. In the IVF process it must be destroyed. In natural procreation the child is conceived and received 'for better or for worse'; in the IVF programme only conditionally – 'for better'.

26. Taking things as they are, knowing the present climate of opinion and the moral outlook which prevails, and being aware of the interests of researchers in this field, and the guidelines recently published, we must accept – although with regret – the fact that IVF programmes will continue and that 'embryology for its own sake' will be pursued. I say 'with regret' because I cannot see any long-term benefit to mankind in aims and procedures which are radically objectionable on moral grounds: for they all fall short of the respect due to every human being, which should never be a mere means, or even a valuable instrument to be used for the interest and benefit of others or of society, or of science. Morality is the ground of human life. It is my view that our society as a whole, and the social practices which aim at and are directed towards the moral and total well-being and development of its members, cannot be sustained if we relinquish that basic respect for the human individual which I have been expressing as the principle that 'no human being is a piece of property'. The designation 'human being', as we have seen, applies to someone from the beginning of his or her existence at conception until his or her end at death.

52

27. Let us assume that in the future IVF programmes develop further only in the therapeutic context of alleviation of infertility (even though we know that in reality malformed or abnormal embryos are disposed of before transfer). What, in that case, would be socially desirable? What might be recommended, not as the moral ideal but as required by the respect due to the human being? I offer as proposals two principles that might guide future development of social forms of life related to human procreation:

(i) The well-being of the child must be of paramount importance; it must be recognised that the child is not a commodity, a piece of property.
(ii) The truth about the child's origins must be communicated confidentialy to the parents (a requirement which does not exclude the preservation of confidentiality); and the responsibility of those contributing to the conception of the child (whether genetically or otherwise) must be guaranteed by whatever means are possible.

Let us consider these two principles in turn.

(1) *The well-being of the child.* The child must be brought into existence for his own sake, 'for better or for worse'. This is a very basic demand of all human beings, of all of us: to be loved and respected for our own sakes and not for any instrumental gains which others may seek from us. In our society a child tends to be thought of merely as an object that satisfies a need. If desired, anything will be done to have it; if not desired it will be rejected, even to the point of being destroyed. This attitude of regarding children as commodities will be fostered by IVF programmes. But what we cannot in fact permit is the commercialisation of human generation that such an attitude may bring with it. Thus, the generative procedures by which a child is brought into existence must not be commercialised. The marketing of sperm and ova and of embryos – through embryo banks – and womb leasing, etc., must all be prohibited. If gametes are donated, this must be done without any financial inducements. 'Generation' is related to 'generosity', to the 'giving' of life which is freely received and must be freely given. If the child is to be brought into existence for

his own sake, procedures for the selection of children on eugenic grounds, or for the moulding of their features and characters according to the interests of political parties, governments or science, must all be excluded. Who are those parties to sit in judgement to determine the course of life of others? Children are not commodities designed to satisfy needs. They claim respect, care and responsible acceptance *as equals* with us.

(2) *Truth and social responsibility.* Bearing in mind the well-being of the child, I cannot subscribe to the so-called 'principle of anonymity'.[45] This is the principle governing artificial insemination by donor (AID), whereby the donor of sperm is anonymous, so that his identity is not disclosed to relatives, the parents or the child himself. Such anonymity breeds irresponsibility. The donor, usually a medical student, is paid £7 per sample of seminal fluid and thereafter has no further responsibility.[46] Why, in AID or other forms of generation, should the child be deprived of knowing who his genetic parents are? Why are we to deprive him of the truth? Why should any action for which we are responsible – if it is a morally good action, or (e.g.) something voluntarily done as an act of generosity to communicate life – always be kept anonymous? To base social relations – relations between doctors, donors and parents, as well as family and other interpersonal relations – on a refusal to disclose the truth and to hold people responsible for their actions is to build our society on shaky foundations. Thus we must secure the confidential disclosure of full information about donors, the removal of all financial inducements for their donations, and the introduction of regulations governing both their rights and their responsibilities.

28. My general recommendation, based both on moral and on social grounds, is that we should strive to encourage adoption rather than generation of human beings by risky technological means which ultimately involve the direct destruction of some human beings. We owe a living to those children already existing. We do not owe a living to those who have not yet come into existence.

29. I also recommend that we continue to support the commitment of our society to research and study, encouraging all proper means of alleviating human suffering. Scientific research should be addressed more directly to questions of *root causes* and of *prevention*[47] which do not involve the direct use and destruction of human beings. Indeed, a continuous effort is demanded of us to support means of alleviating such causes of human suffering as genetic diseases, malformations, other forms of disease and human infertility, as well as the malnutrition and hunger that affects our world. And whether these forms of human suffering occur naturally or whether they result from our unjust dealings with one another, we should be committed to preventing them and to abolishing their real and ultimate causes. The medical and scientific aims and procedures expressing such a commitment can indeed be in accord with the respect owed to every human being, or can be reorientated in that direction. I do not believe that reorientating our means and ends in this direction amounts to abandoning possibilities of progress. It certainly does not imply bringing our research to a standstill. It means looking in other directions to discover new possibilities not previously foreseen because not previously considered. Nature, our powers of intelligence and the true generosity of our minds and hearts will not let us down in this task. In 1969 Dr Edwards said that his research with human embryos would help, among other things, in the discovery of the causes of Down's syndrome with a view to preventing it.[48] It is well known that Professor Lejeune's work in this particular field has been of enormous significance and value. I should like to take his work as an example of that commitment to research and to the progress of science and humanity which we must endorse: tirelessly undertaken and pursued, and with the unconditional respect which is due to every human being from the beginning of his or her existence.

30. Let me finish on a note of hope. Moral issues can only be sorted out and tackled by moral means and with moral courage. There is no other solution for them than our moral strength. That key and that power is within each one of us. So there is always hope. Recently I saw the following lines being

applied to our policies of nuclear disarmament;[49] they can be applied also to our present topic. They summarise much of what I have been trying to say here:

> Point not the goal, until you plot the course,
> For ends and means to man are tangled so
> That different means quite different aims enforce;
> Conceive the means as ends in embryo.

3

IVF: The basic issue

I. Major issues

1. One of the fundamental critical comments that Professor Mitchell makes in his contribution to the recent *Journal of Medical Ethics* symposium[1] on *in vitro* fertilisation (IVF) is that consideration of the well-being of the child to be brought into existence by artificial methods of reproduction does not feature prominently in Professor Singer's and Mr Wells's discussion. In his reply Professor Singer seeks to rectify this impression and clarifies their position which, he says, 'rests solidly on utilitarian foundations' and 'naturally' – he adds – 'in making our utilitarian calculations, the interests of the potential child must also be taken into account'. It emerges that consideration of the well-being of the child is far from being an overriding factor in the utilitarian calculation. Even if the children generated in an artificial way will be subject to disadvantages directly attributable to that mode of generation, as long as these disadvantages are not so serious 'as to make their lives so miserable as not to be worth living' we may proceed with this mode of generation. Singer goes on to claim that it would require distinctively high suicide rates to show that 'these children do not find their lives worth living'.

Singer's only way of envisaging the good of the child, as it is relevant to determining the acceptability of IVF (in whatever context) and surrogate motherhood, is by way of answer to the question: Would children conceived and reared in these ways get sufficient *satisfaction* out of life to prevent them from committing suicide? It is clear that he lacks any objective

57

conception of the values and goods which make for authentic human development and therefore any conception of normative conditions conducive to fostering those values and goods. The child enters the utilitarian calculation simply as one among a number of potential points at which desires are satisfied. If, like Singer, you imagine yourself able to predict a surplus of satisfied over unsatisfied desires in the life of that child, then there is nothing to count against satisfying another person's desire to have that child.

2. Apart from (i) the well-being of the child-to-be, the other issues discussed in the symposium which I take to be major are (ii) the family as a natural structure of human life (as natural as language), its relation to marriage and to the different forms of artificial parenthood, and (iii) the nature of the human embryo. Other questions, such as the allocation of resources (and the neglected question of infertility) I take to be directly related to the general issue of the ultimate aims of medicine. In my view the essential aim of medicine is the restoration to health (or some approximation of health) of those diseased or impaired, and not the satisfaction of other needs (least of all 'needs' for which our only evidence is strong desire). On Professor Singer's conception of need there can surely be no rational way of settling problems of resource allocation.

3. Professor Mitchell gives full consideration to the essential social dimension of the issues, particularly to the family founded on the marriage covenant as the natural context of generation. He indicates the way in which our society would be deleteriously affected if we were to follow the views and recommendations of Singer and Wells. I share his point of view and believe that to be married is a fundamental condition for assuming the responsibilities of procreation, and that this is not – in moral terms – a mere matter of attitude, as we are told. That Professor Singer's and Mr Wells's views 'are likely to obtain a great deal of support from medical scientists and medical practitioners' is a fact too obvious to require emphasis; it shows the extent to which the prevailing medico-scientific ideology and practice have become utilitarian.

4. Nevertheless, it is not the case, either in theory or in practice or as a matter of tradition, that utilitarianism – in its variety of forms – is the only way or the best way to evaluate and solve our moral and social problems. Indeed, there are alternatives to the utilitarian mentality which are worth considering. My purpose here is to present one briefly. My contribution will centre on the issue which I take to be basic and which deserves closer attention than was given to it in the symposium. It is an issue on which most of the other moral and social issues raised by IVF depend: the nature of the human embryo.

5. There are two routes that I must follow in order to tackle the problems: they can be called the *moral* and the *ontological*. The former route issues in recognition of the values belonging to things, values which govern our behaviour and command our respect; such values as belong to things establish their *moral status*. The latter route issues in recognition of the nature of things – what they are or what the facts show of their mode of being – their *ontological status*. These two routes are interrelated, for we need to know what things are if we are to decide how we should treat them, and the kind of respect owing to them.

II. The moral evaluation

6. What kind of respect is due to the human embryo? We cannot answer this question without first giving an answer to another one: what kind of respect is due to the developed human being or human person? The most basic reply we must give to this latter question may be framed in a simple principle: *no human being is property* – or (what amounts to the same thing) *no human being may be treated as property*. That some human beings have been regarded and/or treated as property by other human beings is both an historical and a current fact.

7. Historically, slavery best illustrates the point. The social institution of slavery made one human being, as a matter of law and practice, the property of another human being. The slave had no claim over his or her life and liberty. He could be used, exploited or even killed and so his life was of purely

59

instrumental value. A slave, both in his life and powers, was radically a means to the interests and benefits of his master. Currently, some have argued that infants (and even young children) are the property of their parents. So parents have the right to dispose of them if such action is deemed desirable or beneficial. It is claimed that children do not have equal moral status to the fully-developed human being, so they can be used for the benefit of others, as in medical experiments; to this kind of end they can be generated and subsequently disposed of. If children are property then they can be treated as property.

The abolition of slavery for every human being – including children – may be taken as one of the greatest steps in the moral development of the human family. It amounts to the recognition of the fundamental moral equality of all human beings. Indeed, human beings are not bits of property, objects or instruments of use to serve the benefits and interests of others. 'No human being is property' is a moral premise of our contemporary society which expresses an egalitarian vision of man, attained through long social struggle and by the suffering lives and deaths of many individual human beings.

8. Recognising the radical equality of status of all members of the human family leads us also to recognise what might be meant by the principle of 'respect for persons'. This respect is a fundamental requirement of justice, in virtue of which no human being is to be used or exploited for any purpose whatsoever. It is a recognition that individually every human being at least has the right not to be used merely as a means to the needs or interests of others and that every innocent human being has at least the right not to be killed. 'Not to be used, not to be killed' is the ultimate moral ground where the roots of justice lie. So it is the point of departure for our dealings with one another in all the social contexts and social forms of life in which we find ourselves and which we continuously create.

9. The moral equality proper to all members of the human family not only pervades our international declarations and bills of rights: it is also enshrined in our laws which are

designed to guarantee and protect the inviolable status of every individual human being. The equality of humans is central to the moral vision of the medical profession, in its attempt to serve life, as expressed in its codes of practice. The paramount value of each human being and the consequent moral necessity to respect him also constitutes a cornerstone or first principle of traditional moral philosophies (the Kantian one being an example) as well as a cornerstone of religious moral thinking and life – as in the Jewish-Christian tradition, for example. Yet for the utilitarian tradition respect for the individual human being is not the paramount moral value; the paramount moral value is rather the realisation of some overall 'best outcome', to achieve which values and persons may be sacrificed. Accordingly, if the circumstances seem to require it, the life or lives of individual human beings may be regarded as instrumental and as expendable for that 'greater good'. Ultimately, in utilitarianism, all values, and individual human beings themselves, can be 'traded off'. This is not so for the kind of non-utilitarian outlook that I want to present. In this outlook any 'calculations' or weighing and comparing of values occurs only on the presupposition that absolute respect for each individual human being is under no circumstances to be 'traded off', that is, that directly harming or destroying innocent human life is never justifiable. In this perspective all human beings are to be treated as morally equal.

10. Yet some non-utilitarians may ask: 'Are all human beings really equal? Are we not to distinguish between the newly-conceived human being – or the "potential human being" or "potential person" – and the fully-developed human being, in full exercise of his or her personal capacities?'.

Professor Singer and Mr Wells claim in their discussion that they 'regard the 1, 2, 4, 8, 16, or 32 cell zygote as not in the same category as a developed human being'. This means that zygotes do not deserve the same moral respect as that accorded to the developed human being, since they are not the same kind of beings. The zygote and the developed human being differ in nature, that is, in their ontological status, hence they differ in their moral status as well. Is this really so? To this question I now turn.

61

III. The nature of the human embryo: development into a person or development of a person?

11. When philosophers and scientists study the nature of things they do so by paying attention to their material (or bodily) configuration, to their behaviour and to the powers and capacities they manifest. In other words, they find out what specific things *are* by how they are materially constituted and by what they do (i.e., their powers and activities). So if we wanted to know about the nature of the human zygote, that is, what the human zygote really *is*, it would not help us to characterise it merely as 'genetic material' or 'biological material' (to use Singer's and Wells's phraseology, now very much used by the medical profession as well), or as something having merely 'biological life'. These expressions do not specify the particular nature of the thing they refer to. By 'genetic material' we could equally mean a segment of DNA, or some of the genes, or all of the chromosomes, or whole germ cells like sperm and the unfertilised ovum, or the zygote. By 'biological material' we could mean all the above plus any somatic cell or group of cells, or organs or even the living being as a whole. The attempt to reduce the human embryo to living material of no specific kind is both scientifically and philosophically incorrect. Let us remember as well that there is no such thing as 'biological life', for life strictly speaking only occurs, is sustained and transmitted in and through *individuals*; and individuals are always of *specific* kinds. There is, doubtless, a pragmatic advantage in describing the newly-conceived human being as 'biological' or 'genetic material'; by a mere device of language you can make it seem that there is nothing wrong in using, experimenting on, destroying, freezing and disposing of embryos – which are just 'material'.

12. So if we are to discern the nature of the zygote we cannot do it by reducing it to mere biological material; we need to know what particular kind of material being the zygote is by its characteristic elements: physical constitution, organisation, inner powers and capacities. We can learn much from the biological sciences in this respect. It is undeniable that 'the embryo is a living member of the species *homo sapiens*' – as

Professor Singer states.[2] But it should be noted, first, that the expression '*homo sapiens*' is not 'neutrally scientific' and bereft of the significant moral implications that some resist in the word 'human'; and secondly, that from a scientific viewpoint a zygote is indeed a new item in the human species, something which is not true of other cells of the human body.

13. The fact that the zygote or embryo is a living human being from conception onwards is, in the view of many people, a sufficient reason to recognise that it must be treated and protected not as property but as a member of the human family. It must be respected in accordance with its particular life-stage and condition; it must not be killed, it must not be used, instrumentalised or exploited for any purpose whatsoever. For many, including Singer and Wells, to be a human being, that is, a member of the human species, does not carry with it any claim on others to respect one's life. What carries this claim is the fact that a human being is in a sufficiently developed state (i.e., is a person) to be able to make this claim as an expression of his or her *desire* to be so respected. Perhaps the two contrasting positions could be clarified in the following terms. The continuity of our existence as human beings, that is, as members of the human species from our earliest embryonic beginnings, could be described as a dynamic process of becoming what we potentially are. This process, though, can be interpreted in two different ways: (a) as the process of development *into* a person, or (b) as the process of development *of* a person. The basic difference between these two interpretations lies in what the term 'potentially' is really taken to involve and in what is ultimately valued in human beings. Let me consider these two positions in turn.

14. (a) *Development into a person*. In this approach it is maintained that we become persons, and may cease to be persons, while our existence as human beings persists all the time. Two unavoidable questions arise: (i) In virtue of what are we to be considered as persons?; and (ii) At what stage of our development as human beings do we become persons?
(i) Philosophers in the tradition of Locke say that a person is an organism possessing 'the concept of self as a continuing

63

subject of experiences and other mental states, and believes that it is itself such a continuing entity'.[3] In brief, self-consciousness and what goes with it is what constitutes us as persons. Within this perspective, what is valued in human beings, i.e., that which leads us to believe that they have moral claims upon us, is the actual exercise of capacities associated with self-consciousness. It should be noted that the moral claims upon us even of fully-fledged persons are from this point of view not held to be absolute; for specific claims upon us (that is, rights which imply correlative obligations) are not based on the simple fact of 'personhood'; rather they are based on the *expressed desires* of persons, which may change. So the right a person may have not to be killed can be waived if he desires to be killed. Personhood is itself not valuable; what is ultimately valuable about being a person is that you have reached that stage of development at which, having the required conceptual equipment, you are in a position to express that range of desires, satisfaction of which is alone morally significant. (Animals are capable of expressing their desires, such as the desire not to suffer pain, as much as humans are; hence, in this view, they also have rights based on those desires; they have moral claims upon us.)

(ii) Those adhering to these views maintain that the particular moment at which a human being becomes a person, i.e., turns into a person by acquiring a concept of self and a range of other concepts necessary to having and expressing desires, is a matter for empirical determination. This determination can be left to the psychologists and is relatively unproblematic.

15. (b) *Development of a person.* In this approach, in contrast to the previous one, to be a human being is to be a person. There are no stages in our existence at which this identity does not hold. If this is so, the concept of a person cannot be determined by, or restricted to, a stage – or state – of self-consciousness. Thus, within this outlook also there are two questions which must be answered: (i) If what makes someone a person is not self-consciousness, and the belief that one is a continuing self, what is it?; and (ii) If fundamental rights (and obligations) are not based on conscious desires, on what are they based, and how are they related to personhood?

(i) What makes us persons is the *kind of beings we are*, the kind of nature we possess, and not a passing state or stage of that kind of being. I shall undertake to make good these claims in the light of two principles which for convenience may be called *the principle of unity* and *the principle of potentiality*. By the principle of unity is meant that a human being – like any other creature – is just one entity, one being, and not a composite of two things. It is not first a physical organic body with (at a later stage) personhood added to it by self-consciousness, making it a human being *and* a person. It is not a human organism first and a person only subsequently, in virtue of the advent of a 'soul' or consciousness. Human beings are what they are on the basis of their specific organic make-up, with its proper constitution, powers and activities. Both our organism and our powers are inseparably one and of a specific kind, of a 'human' kind, we say: that is why we call ourselves 'human' beings. Our organic make-up, in its molecular structure (the human genes) as well as in its bodily form (the human face and hands, the human brain and feet, the human eyes) are not something separable from, or something capable of being abstracted from, the powers they express and realise, powers whose exercise *is* what living consists in as far as we are concerned: eating, drinking, sleeping, movement from place to place, smiling, laughing, speaking a language, hoping, being open- or narrow-minded, pursuing ends, choosing means, adopting attitudes, determining the course of one's life. It has been rightly noted that when the idea of consciousness is completely separated from, abstracted from, humanity and human life, philosophers develop two typical syndromes, of which one is 'a dire suspicion that anything at all may be a subject of consciousness',[4] e.g., animals or a brain *in vitro*. We appropriately consider ourselves to be part of the animal kingdom because of our bodily condition. Yet our bodily condition is not something apart from what we distinctively are, with all our powers and activities, including self-consciousness, self-determination, responsibility, love and creativity. Because of all these, we see ourselves as different from other creatures and regard ourselves as persons. We acknowledge that we are the only beings that, because of our human body and powers, live and respond to reality and to others in a

65

personal way. It is also in virtue of what we are as a unity of body and pow:rs and activities that we regard ourselves as belonging to one and the same family, one and the same species, long described as *homo sapiens*. Members of this species manifest their *personal* form of life not only individually but also socially. We are the only creatures that live culturally, that manifest their higher form of life in the so-called universals of culture, namely, linguistic activity, conscience, art and aesthetic appreciation, religion, political life and technology. Indeed bodily form (or organic form) and powers are the two inseparable dimensions and determinants of any species, of any members of the animal kingdom, making them what they are in their specific nature. What things can do and how they appear is a manifestation of what they are. It is what they are that determines what they can do, not the other way round. So if we can attain self-consciousness at some stage, we must *already* be the kind of beings that can attain it.

The inseparability of what a thing is and its powers is particularly manifested in its organic continuity, in its being always the same organism. This question of continuity leads us to the principle of potentiality. The bodily person I am now certainly began as a tiny organism of one cell, a human zygote. If this original cell was capable of developing into *me*, what powers and potential did it have then? This is the crucial question that must be answered. The development of personal abilities (self-awareness, choice, creativity) does not come about independently of our organic development. There is no basis in reality for affirming that those powers are 'something added' (by miracle?) at any particular stage. Thus if we are to make sense of our existence *now* as human personal beings, we must admit that whatever powers we have now have developed from the ones we had at the beginning. Our present abilities are explicable only if the immanent power for those abilities was always present in the human organism right from the beginning. To say that only at some later stage of development do we have the *exercisable* abilities of self-consciousness and self-determination, while true, leaves unexplained the origin and development of these abilities; and failure to recognise the need for explanation at this point results in failure to acknowledge the nature of the *subject* to which the abilities belong. The value of a being is indeed related to the things into which it can develop, not independently of, but precisely because of what the being is. For the actual power to achieve a particular type of development must always have been present prior to the development, and is therefore significant in determining what kind of being we are dealing with, even in the earliest stages of its existence.

16. We know that a new human individual organism with the internal power to develop into an adult, given nurture, comes into existence as a result of the process of fertilisation at conception. We must reckon then that such a power is an actually present source of potentialities which in the normal course of development will come to be more or less fully manifested in the personal life of an adult. Hence, the kind of life that the zygote has, because of the power it presently possesses, is personal life, that is, the life of a personal being or a personal subject. It is this presence of personal powers – which must be attributable to a personal subject – that makes a difference between one kind of life (that of human persons) and another (that of, say, dogs). It must also be noted that living entities are not machines built up out of blocks. The development of a living entity, its becoming what it is capable of being, is indeed a process, but the entity itself and its coming-to-be are not. At any particular time, the entity is *in toto* or it is not at all (this is an important consideration for the debate about brain death as well; see below, Chapter Six, para. 16–22). For living human beings are not like (for example) clocks, that progressively come to be and can be assembled and dismantled. Whereas you can reasonably speak of having half a clock, you cannot reasonably speak of having half a person.

(ii) Let us now turn to the question of basic rights. It is in virtue of what things are that we treat them one way or another; it is in virtue of what human beings are, right from the beginning of their existence, that they must be accorded absolute respect and their lives treated as inviolable. Rights are based on values, and values on the recognition of what things are. The ultimate ground of value is being, not transitory states of beings, like activities and desires; for these are the manifestations of what the being is. What one can become is a possibility based on what one is. Becoming has its only basis in being. Every potentiality must be based on something actual, on a power which is really present. Basic rights (and obligations), such as the right not to be killed and the obligation not to kill an innocent human being, are based on what human beings are, not on particular states of conscious desires. Thus from this perspective what is valued in human beings is *themselves*, what they are, and not just what they achieve.

IV. What is morally desirable

17. In the strict sense the problem of IVF is not a medical problem, one which arises from concern for health and the development of means to restore or improve health; for the procedure is aimed at fulfilling the desire to have a child. Rather it is one of an increasing number of biotechnical problems, that is, problems arising from the development of techniques designed to circumvent or modify existing (usually defective) modes of bodily function. These biotechnical developments along with other scientific developments 'threaten to turn *homo sapiens* into *homo mechanicus*', as has recently been noted.[5] Although this is a general point, it is one of great significance in relation to the direction medicine is now taking. It cannot be ignored in our evaluations of medical progress and development.

18. Having said that, I wish now to turn to our main question. What kind of respect is due to the human embryo? Is the human embryo to be protected as a human being or as property? The only possible answer, in the light of the considerations advanced in the previous section, is that the respect due to the human embryo must not differ in kind from the respect due to any other adult human being; the human embryo, because it is a human being, must be protected as a human being, not as a property or an object of use. This means that the human embryo has the right not to be killed and not to be used or exploited for any purpose whatever.

This makes it clear that a form of study which risks harm to human embryos and experimentation on human embryos for scientific purposes is immoral. Such experiments are never in the interest of the subject experimented upon, who is harmed, used up and destroyed, always being treated radically as a means, as an object of use, as a 'product', as 'material' – to use favourite dehumanising terms in vogue in the literature.

19. In the context of alleviating infertility, a number of spare embryos are generated, this being the most economic procedure for attaining the general aim in view – the best possible chance of pregnancy with a minimum of effort, expense and trauma. Yet the well-being and existence of each individual human being thus generated is made secondary and as such instrumental to the general aim. Those human lives, if not required for the desired pregnancy, will be disposed of, used for experiments, or frozen until a time comes when they will be in demand for implantation, experimentation or disposal. The common practice of superovulation clearly involves an immoral instrumentalisation of the embryo.

20. We are told that nature 'prodigally' disposes of large numbers of embryos, even without this being noticed by the women who carry them. Hence, some ask, if nature is so prodigal with so many embryos, why are we not entitled to generate some that can be used for the benefit of others or of science, and, when necessary, destroyed or disposed of? First, it should be remarked that even if it were true that many embryos die naturally, that fact would tell us nothing about what kind of being the embryo is, or, therefore, about what kind of respect is owed to it. Secondly, natural processes such as floods, droughts, volcanic eruptions and other kinds of natural disasters are natural processes as much as the processes whereby the loss of fertilised ova naturally occur. These processes cannot be taken as indicative of what we are to do, of the actions we are to choose. To think otherwise is to ignore the fact that what we intend, decide and deliberately bring about are not, in this sense, natural processes (and just because they are not, we are answerable for them). Hence they cannot be measured against the results that nature brings about. We are moral beings. Physical nature is not.

21. Irreparable damage to the embryo or the child-to-be is a feature of IVF procedures which cannot be excluded. This is clearly acknowledged by (for example) Dr Edwards, when he mentions the back-up methods of monitoring abnormalities after IVF and implantation, and suggests *in vitro* abortion.[6] This risk is implicitly recognised in the report on IVF by the Royal College of Obstetricians and Gynaecologists in Great Britain, when it claims that the 'possibility that a child born with an abnormality might in due course be able to sue its parents and the doctors cannot be ruled out'.[7] We are not morally justified in directly engaging in bringing about such risk of harm. In natural procreation an abnormal embryo might or might not abort. In the IVF process it must be destroyed. In natural procreation the child is conceived and received unconditionally 'for better or for worse', but in the IVF programme only conditionally and 'for better', and so primarily not for his or her own sake but for the satisfaction of a desire. It needs to be recognised that the well-being of the child should be of paramount importance – as that of any other human being; recognition of this should be embodied in attitudes and practices which exclude treating the child as a commodity, a property or a mere object of satisfaction at any stage of his or her existence.

22. One should welcome the fact that Singer and Wells recognise that secrecy over gamete donation (as may occur in artificial insemination by donor (AID) or in surrogate motherhood) need not be maintained. Openness will indeed encourage greater responsibility and attitudes of trust and truth in all those involved. Yet meeting the requirements of openness hardly answers all the objections to these practices. Not only do the practices put the well-being of the child at risk, but surrogate motherhood, in particular, involves a direct instrumentalisation of the feminine power of gestation. The phrase 'rent-a-womb' fairly aptly characterises the instrumentalisation in question; for whether one pays or not, the woman's body becomes usable accommodation. Neither children born or unborn, nor women, nor the rest of mankind are ever to be property, but beings to be respected, cared for and

loved for their own sake, and not with a view to achieving other purposes. We all have to grow in that rare virtue that men of great stature have shown: to love human beings just because they are human beings.

4

The human being and the right not to be killed

I. A controversial distinction:
'human beings' and 'human persons'

1. Any particular moral stance reflects a particular evaluation of the human individual, resting on certain presuppositions about the kind of being a human individual is. For the obligations we owe to human beings, and hence the rights we regard them as possessing, are ultimately dependent upon what we take human beings to be and on the worth we acknowledge them to have. Now there are some who maintain that to be a human being is not necessarily to be a human person; that not all human beings are persons and not all persons need be human beings. In ordinary everyday life, people use the terms 'human being' and 'human person' to refer to the same range of beings, and the ordinary use of the term 'person' is such that all human beings count as persons.[1] Nevertheless, some contemporary philosophers would claim that the tendency to use expressions like 'person' and 'human being' interchangeably is not always justified.[2] They claim that because we fail to see that not all human beings are persons, we mistakenly attribute basic rights (such as the right to life) to all human beings, whereas in their view it is only persons (a restricted subclass of human beings) who properly enjoy basic rights; it is only someone who is truly a person who has the right not to be killed. Hence proponents of this view state that the key question is: 'What makes something a person and what gives something the right not to be killed?' It must be noted that there are two questions here, and that the

answer to the first is taken as the basis for the answer to the second.

2. The drawing of a distinction between the meaning of the terms 'human being' and 'human person' is a recent development. In the Western philosophical tradition it can be traced to certain sixteenth-century philosophers. The concept of a person itself entered into philosophical discussion in mediaeval times, by way of theology.[3] The roots of the 'human being'/'human person' distinction may be found in a form of empiricism (ultimately dualistic in its implications) of which the philosopher Locke is a representative exponent. In his *Essay Concerning Human Understanding*, Book II, Chapter XXVII, Locke characterises a person as 'a thinking intelligent being, that has reason and reflection, and can consider itself as itself . . . which it does only by that consciousness which is inseparable from thinking'. A human person described in these terms is the adult human person who possesses self-consciousness, is a subject of moral obligations, is therefore morally accountable for his or her actions – both to his or her conscience and to others, and, sometimes, before a court of law. But this moral/legal description of the meaning of the term 'person' excludes infants and those with some kind of brain injury or deficiency who cannot be described as 'reasoning and reflective'.

3. In the classic (non-empiricist and non-dualist) European philosophical tradition, which accords with people's ordinary common-sense outlook, any human being who is born and who looks, lives and behaves like us is a person. The human being is not reduced to his or her actual reasoning powers. Rather, to be a human being is to be a being of a particular physical constitution, of a particular bodily nature, namely, that of the species *homo sapiens*, endowed with the powers proper to that human nature, even when (because of immaturity or old age, or because there has been an organic bodily injury or some other deficiency) these powers cannot be expressed or manifested or exercised. If to be a human person is something over and above being 'merely' a human being, then the bodily being – that which is sometimes said to possess

'mere biological life' – may be regarded as a kind of instrument or machine used by a reasoning 'I' who is (on this view) the real person; so that when the ability to reason goes the person goes, and what is left behind is mere biological life.

4. Let me focus first on what is not in dispute: that the adult human being who is a knowing subject with a certain degree of freedom for self-determination is certainly a person. No-one doubts that whoever is an autonomous free agent, and therefore a subject responsible for his actions, is a person. To recognise the human person as an autonomous and responsible agent is to recognise him as a subject of rights and obligations. He is a subject of rights because, being autonomous and responsible, he deserves to be treated as such by others; and he is a subject of obligations or duties because he too has to treat others in accordance with what is owed to them as responsible and autonomous subjects. To say this is to recognise that although human persons are bodily organisms and share certain characteristics with other living creatures and artifacts – they are, for example, all subject to physical laws such as that of gravity – they are not totally determined by either physical or biological laws in choosing ultimate goals for their lives and in acting. Within the framework of the physcial laws to which they are subject, human persons have still the power of exercising freedom and responsibility.

5. It is also undisputed that our individual histories as bodily human beings had an organic beginning, encompassing certain stages of development, and will have an end in death. There is an undeniable continuity in our organic development: every one of us has been a zygote, an embryo and then a foetus, an infant and a child, and has then passed through different stages of development to adulthood and maturity. There are no relevant 'cut-off points' as regards our existence as human beings, just as there are no such 'cut-off points' in the existence of other animals. This continuity of existence as human beings from our early beginnings could be described as an inner process of becoming in actual fact what we are potentially all along. It is clear that the embryonic being, once it is generated, contains actual immanent powers which permit it

74

to become the adult through a continuous process of development.

6. There are two different approaches to recognising the significance and implications of this continuous process of development of the embryonic human being to adulthood. The first approach involves claiming that although there is a biological or organic continuity in the existence of the being (making it at all stages a human being, a member of the human species), there is no corresponding *personal* continuity, no continuity of existence as a personal being. It is maintained, then, that we come to be persons and that we may cease to be persons even though our existence as human beings persists. Hence there are stages when we are human beings but not persons. The second approach denies this position by maintaining that the generated bodily being of human kind, the human being, is always a human person.

II. Human desires and human rights

7. The first approach inevitably provokes the question: Given that there is organic continuity in the development of the human being from its very beginnings, at what stage of this development does the human being become a person, and in virtue of what does he or she become a person? In order to answer this question let me take Michael Tooley's position as representative of this first approach.[4] Tooley, following Locke, says that a person is an organism which possesses 'the concept of self as a continuing subject of experiences and other mental states, and believes that it is itself such a continuing entity'. Note the two requirements involved: possession of the concept of self; belief that the concept applies in one's own case. On this view it is the actual exercisable capacity of self-consciousness that constitutes personhood. Other philosophers[5] consider that the minimum requirement for personhood is sentience, the capacity to feel, that is actualised when the nervous system begins to appear; this nervous system, with its centre in the brain, is the basis for the actualisation of self-consciousness. In both cases, what is valued in human beings, i.e., that which is considered the basis for treating

human beings with respect, is the actual exercisable capacity for self-awareness. Nevertheless, this value has no adequate moral significance directly in itself, for Tooley tells us that 'rights are not founded on values': the right not to be killed (for example) is not founded on the fact that human beings are persons, beings possessing the exercisable power of self-consciousness. Rather, rights are ultimately founded on what persons (or indeed animals) *desire*. That is why 'A has a right to X' is roughly synonymous with 'If A desires X, then others are under a *prima facie* obligation to refrain from actions that would deprive him of it'. It is said to follow from this that if an individual asks someone to destroy something to which he has a right, that other does not violate the individual's right to that thing if he proceeds to destroy it – even if it happens to be the individual's own life. For if the individual ceases to desire X (if he ceases, for example, to desire to keep on living) he ceases to have a right to X, and the other ceases to have the obligation to preserve or respect X.

8. Thus the right to life, that is, the right not to be killed, is considered to belong to a person not just because he or she is a person, but rather in virtue of the desire that that person has to continue to live. Now it is argued that someone can desire to continue to live as the person he or she is only if he or she (i) possesses a concept of the self and (ii) thinks of himself or herself as a self capable of continued existence. Both (i) and (ii) are said to be essential to possessing self-conscious awareness, and it is self-conscious awareness which (in the tradition of Locke) makes one a person.

9. The underlying ethical viewpoint here is that morality is concerned with the satisfaction of desires. But because not all desires can be satisfied, the rights which are founded on desires entail no more than *prima facie* obligations, that is, obligations which may be overridden by other claims upon us. Moreover, as obligations are relative to rights, and rights to desires, and desires come and go, are present or absent, our obligations towards others are conditional. Our obligations towards them are fundamentally to give them what they want, or at least not to prevent them from obtaining it for themselves.

10. Philosophers adhering to this view maintain that the particular moment at which a human being becomes a person, that is, turns into a person by coming to have a concept of self and a desire to continue to live as a self, is a matter for empirical determination. Such determination is left to psychologists and is held not to give rise to any serious practical difficulties. Tooley says:

> There is no serious need to know the exact point at which a human infant acquires a right to life. For in the vast majority of cases in which infanticide is desirable, its desirability will be apparent within a short time after birth.

III. Human nature and human rights

11. An alternative approach to the one just discussed is based on the recognition that the human being is always a person because the concept of person cannot be determined merely by, or be restricted to, a stage (or state) of self-consciousness. Also, and because of this, rights are not to be founded on self-conscious desires, and so they are not necessarily connected with states of consciousness. Within this outlook two questions must be answered. First, what is it that makes someone a person if it is not self-consciousness?; and secondly, if fundamental rights and obligations are not based on conscious desires, on what are they based, and how are they related to personhood?

12. What makes us persons is the kind of beings we are, our human nature, and not a conscious state or passing stage in the life of that kind of being. Let us consider how we may come to recognise what we are. Human beings are single entities, each one is just one being, as other animals are also. Human beings are what they are in virtue of (a) their specific organic constitution with its proper structure, and (b) their specific powers which result from this organic constitution and which manifest themselves in specific activities.

13. Our bodily organism, and the powers that belong to it, are inseparably one and of a specific kind – of human kind, as we say: that is why we call ourselves *human* beings. Our organic

make-up, in its molecular structure (the human genes), as well as in its bodily shape and constitution (the human face, brain and feet, eyes and limbs), are not something separable from, or something capable of being abstracted from, our powers or from the things we do in our everyday lives: eating, drinking, sleeping, moving from place to place, smiling, laughing, yawning, adopting attitudes, determining the course of our lives. We rightly consider ourselves to be part of the animal kingdom because of our bodily condition. Yet our bodily condition is not something apart from what we distinctively are, with all our powers and activities, including the powers of self-consciousness, self-determination, responsibility, love and creativity. Both because of our bodily constitution and because of our various powers and activities we see ourselves as different from other creatures and regard ourselves as persons. We acknowledge that we are the only beings which, while having a specifically human body and powers, live and respond to reality in a personal way.

14. Clearly it is also because each of us is a unity of body, powers and activities that we regard ourselves as belonging to one and the same family, one and the same species, *homo sapiens*, sharing one and the same human nature. Members of this species manifest their personal form of life not only individually but socially. We are the only creatures that live *culturally*, that manifest their nature in the so-called universals of culture, namely, linguistic activity, conscience, art and aesthetic appreciation, religion, political life and technology. Indeed our bodily constitution and powers are what determine the species to which a living creature belongs. They constitute the two inseparable dimensions of every species of the animal kingdom, making them what they are. What beings can do is a manifestation of what they are. It is what they are that determines what they can do, not the other way about. If we can attain self-consciousness at some stage, we must already have been the kind of beings that have the power to attain it. We must emphasise the unity of a living being – the fact that an organism is inseparably one with its powers – if we are not to make the mistake of considering the human organism as something 'biologically neutral', as mere living material of no

relevance to its intrinsic specific organisation, power and activities, which in fact make it what it is: a being of human nature.

15. The inseparability of a thing's physical constitution from its various powers and characteristic activities is manifested particularly in its organic continuity, in its being always the same organism. Let me now consider this point. The bodily person I am now certainly began as a tiny organism of one cell, a human zygote. If this original cell developed into me, *what power did it have* to do so? This is the crucial question that must be answered. The development of personal abilities (self-awareness, choice, affection, creativity) does not come about independently of our organic development. There is no reason for affirming that those powers are something 'added on' at any particular stage. Thus, if we are to make sense of our existence now as human personal beings, we must admit that whatever powers we have now, in virtue of which we do what we do now, are a manifestation or development of the powers we had from the beginning. To say that only at some later stage of development do we have the exercisable powers of self-consciousness and self-determination leaves unexplained the origin, cause and development of these powers and activities, and manifests a failure to acknowlege the nature of the subject to which these abilities belong. The value of a being is indeed related to the things into which it has the power to develop – not independently of, but precisely because of, what the being is. The power to develop into the adult of the species is proper to the nature of the embryo, and this power (together with the actual physical constitution of the embryo) makes it to be the kind of embryo it is and no other. The power may therefore be described as a *constitutional* power, that is, a power making (constituting) the embryo as the kind of being it is. The actual power to achieve a particular type of development must always have been present prior to the development and is therefore significant in identifying what kind of being we are dealing with, even in the earliest stages of its existence.

16. We know that a new individual human organism with the immanent power to develop (given nurture) into an adult

comes into existence at conception, as a result of the process of fertilisation. We must conclude, then, that such a power is something actually present which in the normal course of development will become manifested, more or less fully, in the personal life of an adult. The kind of life possessed by the zygote is, on account of the power it presently possess, personal life, the life of a personal being or a personal subject. It is this presence of personal power, implying as it does the presence of a personal subject, that makes a difference between one kind of embryonic life (that of human persons) and another (that of, say, dogs).

17. Let me now consider the question of basic rights, and in particular the right not to be killed. It is in virtue of what human beings are that their lives are to be respected. Rights, and their corresponding obligations, are based on what we morally value in human beings, and this is ultimately dependent on a recognition of what they truly are. The foundations of moral value (and so of justice) lie in being, in the nature of the human being as such; they are not built on passing states of being such as desires; the latter are simply manifestations of what the human being is (*agere sequitur esse*, as the traditional principle expresses it). What one may become is a function of what one is; every potentiality must be grounded in an actual power. Thus, if we know the potentialities of something we know what that being may in the future become. And the right not to be killed at the very beginning of human life is based on the intrinsic value of the human being, a value related to what the human being essentially is and not merely to particular states of consciousness or desires.

IV. The right not to be killed

18. Ordinarily the term 'the right to life' has the same meaning as the phrase which I am using here, 'the right not to be killed'. There are two reasons for choosing the latter term rather than the former. First, when someone has a right to life he or she is already alive, in existence, living. Therefore the expression 'the right to life' really means something like the following: that one should not interfere with or destroy that life but

80

should rather let it be and allow it to develop. In other words, an assertion of the right to life of human beings means that human beings may not be killed; so the words 'the right not to be killed' bring out the content of this right more explicitly. The effective exercise of this right to life does not arise primarily, therefore, in the individual who possesses it, but in another human being or beings who consider themselves obliged not to kill him or her. In this sense the obligation not to kill is more basic than the right not to be killed. It is precisely with the very recognition of what a human being is that the recognition of the obligation to treat him or her with respect emerges. There are moral dispositions that must be constitutive of the outlook of a person if this recognition is to be really and effectively present. Let me focus first on the basic character of the obligation not to kill a human being.

19. What is due in justice to every human being by the very fact of being a human being? This question has been succinctly answered by the French philosopher Simone Weil in these terms: 'Justice consists in seeing that no harm is done to human beings'.[6] The most basic harm, the most basic wrong, we can do to another human being is to kill him or her. The basic character of the prohibition against killing may be seen in relation to other prohibitions which seek to defend and promote the welfare of human beings, e.g., the prohibitions of stealing, lying, committing adultery, committing sexual assault, and so on. The prohibition of killing is the most basic because it is the precondition of respect for all other aspects of human well-being. All other prohibitions (and obligations, with their corresponding rights) must be kept in order to preserve and foster the goods and values which are aspects of the well-being of human individuals, that is, aspects of the personal integrity and fulfilment of the individual. Yet the obligation not to kill him or her does not make reference merely to aspects of human well-being, but rather to the human individual as such, to his very being in existence. Obligations and considerations of the well-being of a person could not make sense if the person were not first and foremost respected and preserved in existence. In other words, the prohibition of the killing of a human being is basic to the

institution of morality, basic to the conception of justice, and basic to the legal institutions designed for the administration of justice. Unless one recognises the obligation not to kill and hence the prohibition against killing, one can hardly see the force of other prohibitions and obligations which have as their point the well-being of human beings.

20. Considering the obligation not to kill in the context of human beings who are innocent (i.e., who have not made an unjust attack on another), the prohibition of killing must be considered to have an absolute character. There will, then, be an absolute prohibition of murder, for murder, in the moral sense, is the intentional killing of the innocent. To say that the prohibition of killing the innocent is absolute is to say that there are no circumstances in which this prohibition does not hold. The obligation not to kill the innocent, and the corresponding right not to be killed, provides the basis of all justice in our dealings with one another. The absolute character of this obligation has its foundation in the nature of the *subject* of the obligation, who can only be a human being; obligations are binding only on human human beings and not on other animals (even if the latter are considered to be subjects of rights). Also, the *object* of an absolute obligation, in the realm of human affairs, is the human being only. The obligation rests solely on what is perceived to hold true of any human being; hence the obligation is *universal* because it pertains to human beings just because they are human beings. The obligation is therefore a binding one in reference to every human being, whether or not the human being asserts his right not to be killed or is even capable of asserting it.

21. To say that 'the obligation rests solely on what is perceived to hold true of any human being' is to imply that a person who realises that he is under a moral obligation must have a certain *moral attitude* which enables him to perceive this. That moral attitude, and the related capacity to perceive, is characteristic of a truly religious person, that is, a person who has a 'religious sense'. (It is clear that this religious sense is not 'guaranteed' by the fact that one belongs to a particular religious body or denomination, but is rather the result of the moral character of

82

the person himself.) The religious person is capable of recognising an intrinsic worth in every human being, deriving from his mysterious nature and his relationship to a divine origin. However, the recognition of this worth of the human being and the recognition that one is obliged to respect him absolutely are inseparable, and both acts of recognition result from a personal moral attitude. That attitude, as it has been said, is 'the solid foundation for recognising that persons have *rights* to be treated *justly*'.[7] Basic rights, such as the right not to be killed, are recognised, and so made effective by others, but are not granted by them when certain conditions, whether personal or social, are fulfilled. Basic rights are unconditional, and hence are to be respected unconditionally. A basic right is something that is owed to human beings on account of the kind of beings they are.

22. What, then, must be presupposed by those who maintain that one may sometimes be justified in killing the innocent? What justifications could there be that do not undermine the worth of each one of us? How could it be morally acceptable that some human beings can be considered outside the realm of justice and be deliberately wronged? Why some and not others? Any human conscience can be undermined by self-interest or passion and may hence be blind or totally unresponsive to the claims of justice. But the claims are there. In general, the recognition of the personal worth and character of the human being is incompatible with any treatment of human beings which views them *instrumentally*, that is, as expendable in certain circumstances, given certain 'necessities'. 'The real demand of justice is to think of each human being as an end',[8] not as property or as a slave that may be used, exploited and killed in favour of his master's interest.

V. Civil authority and human rights

23. A fundamental task of any government is to protect its members against unjust attacks by others. In other words, the basic rationale for the very existence of civil authority is the protection of those who otherwise would be subject to unjust attack. Hence action sanctioned or carried out by civil

authority which amounts to an attack on the innocent, that is, to an infringement of the right not to be killed, must destroy the legitimacy of civil authority. The laws by which such sanctions are made are unjust laws.

24. The recognition that there are rights naturally due to human beings which the government is obliged to protect is at the very foundations of justice and is necessary if the civil procedures for the administration of justice are to be legitimate. Basic rights are not bestowed by civil authority, but are prior to the civil authority, which must be set up to protect those rights. If civil authority were to engage in violent and unjust attacks on those innocent people whom it is meant to protect, its violence would be different only in name from that of a criminal band.[9]

25. Also, governmental authorisation of the killing of the innocent by other bodies or persons can have no justification. If non-governmental bodies seek or demand of government that killing of the innocent be treated as legitimate (or that it be decriminalised) they are in fact demanding something which destroys the *raison d'être* of civil authority itself. For the very foundation on which authority rests is that human beings have certain basic natural rights, such as the right not to be killed, which need to be protected and championed by civil authority itself.

5

What kind of being is the human embryo?

I. The concept of the human embryo

1. The question 'What kind of being is the human embryo?' contains two main terms: 'kind of being' and 'human embryo'. Use of the first term presupposes that there are a variety of kinds of being, or entity, in reality. One kind of being consists of natural entities like stones or rocks which we call non-living beings, inanimate entities. There are other non-living entities like motor cars and chairs which we describe as artefacts, and some others which we call works of art, such as paintings. These are entities brought about by human design and human hands; they are not products of the natural world itself.

2. Other kinds of natural entity are plants and animals, among which the human being counts as one kind of animal within the various mammalian species. Plants and animals are living beings, animate beings. In these beings what we call 'life' is manifested. The human embryo – as any other animal embryo – counts among the living beings of nature. It is not an inanimate entity, like a rock, or an artefact, like a machine. I shall come to this point later; it is of great importance, although apparently obvious.

3. The human embryo is referred to in a variety of ways in current biomedical literature and in public debate. Let me mention some of the expressions which are used to refer to or to describe it: 'pre-embryo' (a term of quite recent coinage), 'cluster of cells', 'a human biological node', 'human

embryonic material', 'a biological being', 'not a full human', 'a potential human', 'a full human', 'a human being', 'a human personal being', 'a blob of cells', 'the product of conception', 'a conceptus'. What is behind this variety of descriptions – some of them incompatible with others – of one and the same being? It is the question of the true *ontological status* of the human embryo, that is, the question concerning the specific kind of being the human embryo is. By 'human embryo' I understand the human conceptus formed when the process of fertilisation is completed, and persisting through all subsequent stages of development before it acquires an obviously human appearance. After that stage the human conceptus is usually described as a fetus until the time of birth.

The questions, then, which we have to consider are these: Is the human embryo a mere conglomeration of molecules and cells, 'human embryonic material'? Is the human embryo a living human being but not a human person? Is the embryo a living human being and a human person? My conviction is that the human embryo is a human person, a being of human nature with an eternal destiny. I take this conviction to be true, and grounded on biological knowledge, philosophical reflection and the Christian faith and way of life which I share with other Christians in the community we form as a Church. But this conviction is not universally shared. Hence it is my responsibility to witness to it in dialogue and co-operation with Christians and non-Christians alike. This is what we are here for.

4. Our attitude cannot be one of avoiding the issue of the status of the embryo altogether, either because it is difficult or because it does not suit us. People of conscience and integrity have to face difficult questions when they are important. In June 1985 the Board for Social Responsibility of the Church of England issued a Report on Human Fertilisation and Embryology entitled *Personal Origins*. On page 33, section 97 of this report we read:

> However difficult it may be to decide whether the early embryo is, or is not, a human being, in the most important sense of the term, the question to be resolved is still whether something is or is not the case, and not some other kind of question.

In this particular context, 'whether something is or is not the case' means whether the human embryo is a human being in the full sense or not, that is, whether it is or is not 'one of us', a being whose nature is both human and personal. The real question indeed is an ontological question, a question connected with 'being'. The text of *Personal Origins* continues:

> Some of our contemporaries have hoped to avoid the question of the embryo's status altogether, and have thought it possible to move directly to a purely deliberative question: how are we to *act* towards the early embryo? The implication of this manoeuvre would seem to be that human status is not so much discerned as conferred; that social practice is sufficient of itself to validate the claims of any pretence to humanity. The authors of this report . . . are agreed in finding this solution unsatisfactory.

5. So do I. For it is clear that if I do not know what kind of being the human embryo is, neither will I know how I should act towards it. If I do not know for certain what the human embryo really is, then I cannot know what its proper value is, or, therefore, what moral claims it has upon me. It is clear that we need to know what things are if we are to come to know how we should treat them and the kind of respect which we owe them. Questions of 'being' and 'not being' are not mere matters of wilful decision. Rather, they require on our part a sense of human and intellectual responsibility in the recognition and appreciation of what is true independently of our wishes. An attitude of respect for truth, the whole truth, is the necessary precondition for determining questions of what is and what is not, making possible the advancement of true wisdom and knowledge. Michael Polanyi has written in connection with this attitude:

> A man who has learned to respect the truth will feel entitled to uphold the truth against the very society which has taught him to respect it. He will indeed demand respect for himself on the grounds of his own respect for truth, and this will be accepted, even against their own inclinations, by those who share his basic convictions. Such is the equality of men in a free society.[1]

87

II. The *Warnock Report's* question: How is it right to treat the human embryo?

6. The majority of the signatories of the Warnock Report are to be included among those of our contemporaries referred to in *Personal Origins* who have avoided the crucial question concerning the human embryo, namely: Is it or is it not a human person? The Warnock Report states:

> Although the questions of when life or personhood begin appear to be questions of fact susceptible of straightforward answers, we hold that the answers to such questions in fact are complex amalgams of factual and moral judgements. Instead of trying to answer these questions directly we have therefore gone straight to the question of *how it is right to treat the human embryo*. We have considered what status ought to be accorded to the human embryo, and the answer we give must necessarily be in terms of ethical or moral principles. (11.9.)

7. The question 'How is it right to treat the human embryo?' has been answered in the Warnock Report in two ways. Most members of the Warnock Committee considered that it would be right to treat *some* human embryos as mere means for the benefit of other human beings: some human embryos may be bought and sold, possessed and treated as property, harmed, destroyed and disposed of; some human embryos can be generated for the sole purpose of experimentation and then disposed of before day 14. Of course (according to this majority viewpoint on the committee) not all human embryos should be treated this way, for then there would be no test-tube babies, or indeed babies at all; it would be the end of the human species. Why only some should be treated in this way and not others, and which ones are in which group, is really a matter of chance determined by the intentions and interests of the generators.

The second answer found in the Warnock Report as to how it is right to treat the human embryo is given in Dissent Form B signed by three members of the committee, Madeline Carriline, John Marshall and Jean Walker. It is broadly this (although some qualifications would be needed): Every human embryo should be generated with the sole purpose of allowing it to live and develop, to follow its normal course of development; human embryos are not to be deliberately used, harmed and destroyed as mere instruments for the benefit of others; they are not to be generated with a view to their destruction in order to improve techniques of *in vitro* fertilisation or to advance knowledge.

8. The moral principles in the light of which these two different answers are given are not explicitly stated in the report, but they are clearly discernible. The principles are based on the two alternative basic evaluations of the individual human being. These are:

> (a) The individual human being may be harmed or destroyed for the benefit of others. He is of instrumental value; he need not be respected and treated as an end in himself.
> (b) The individual human being is of such intrinsic worth that he may not be deliberately used, exploited, harmed or destroyed for the benefit of others. He is of non-instrumental value; he must be respected and treated as an end and not as a mere means.

The signatories of the majority report profess to accept the general moral principle that the human being is an end in himself and should never be exploited by another human being, but they qualify their acceptance of the principle by saying that it applies 'in almost every case'. The report states:

> Even in compelling medical circumstances the danger of exploitation of one human being by another appears to the majority of us far to outweigh the potential benefits, in almost every case. That people should treat others as means to their own ends, however desirable the consequences, must always be liable to moral objection. (8.17.)

However, it would be no good to you or me if, in the implementation of this principle, we happened to be among the exceptions allowed for by the phrase 'almost every case'.

9. The signatories of the report cannot avoid adopting a position about the kind of being the human embryo is, and here they are all of one accord: the human embryo is *a potential human being*, or a potential human person (see 11.22 and Dissent Form B.3). By this they mean that the human embryo is the kind of being that of itself, given nurture, will develop to a

stage at which everyone will recognise it to be a human person. Put in more simple terms, the signatories mean that whether we like it or not, we all have to recognise that we have been human embryos, human beings of embryonic form. There is no way in which we can deny *this* truth.

10. The committee members differ among themselves on the moral significance they assign to being a 'potential' human being. For the majority of them it is not of much significance at all: the early embryo can be treated as chattel. By contrast Carriline, Marshall and Walker recognise that a being that is regarded as a potential human has a special status in virtue of this potential. They say: 'It is in our view wrong to create something with the potential for becoming a human person and then deliberately destroy it'. They give an illuminating medical analogy to support their view: 'at no stage was a transplant undertaken with the intention that the patient should not survive'.

11. Let me stress the fundamental point I want to make in what I have said. Underlying current medico-scientific trends which support experimentation on human embryos at the expense of their integrity and well-being, there is a valuation of the individual human being which rests on two basic pre-suppositions. The first of these has to do with morality while the second is an ontological presupposition:

(i) The value and interests of science and the rest of society may override the value and interests of the individual human being; the human being is of instrumental value.

(ii) The newly-conceived human, the human embryo, does not enjoy full human status like one of us, for it is not a human being or a human person, but only a potential one.

Clearly, for those who hold that the human being is not of absolute intrinsic worth, whether the human embryo is a full human being or not is not of decisive importance. For even if it were a human being, given pressing needs, it could be deliberately harmed or 'sacrificed' for the benefit of others as a child or adult might be. If innocent human beings can be harmed, killed, 'sacrificed' for others, the human embryo obviously can. To uphold this view that the innocent human being may be deliberately harmed and destroyed is to abolish the basis on which all legal and natural justice rests. If large numbers in our society advocate this view and promote this attitude, there is an enormous need for true moral witness and an effort to counteract that trend. Let us recall that slavery was declared illegal in Britain in 1807 after the bill for its abolition had been introduced in the House of Commons, debated and defeated eleven times.

12. Let me now focus on the second presupposition mentioned above, namely that the human embryo is only a potential human person, and that therefore to harm or destroy it is not to destroy a human person.

Current embryological knowledge about the generation of animals and human beings clearly establishes the fact that a conceptus exists once the process of fertilisation has been completed. We all know that the new human conceptus will grow of itself into the adult being. Why is it, then, that many of our contemporaries do not recognise that we and the conceptus share a common humanity, and that as humanly equal we should all be equally respected? Why is it that the same embryological facts are interpreted in different ways and accorded a different significance? Why is it so difficult for many to recognise that the terms 'human being' and 'human person' are *absolute* terms, that is, that a living being is either human or not human and that you cannot have 'half a human being', 'half a human person', just as you cannot have 'half a dog' (although you can have something which is half a house and is progressively becoming a complete one). Our problems do not lie with embryology books and what they clearly describe. Where do they lie?

13. They may lie with a defective attitude, a lack of respect for the whole truth – as pointed out earlier – but clearly this is not always the case. Some would put it this way: 'Yes, we know we begin as organic beings at conception, but the issue is not whether the human embryo is a human being or not – for it is one – but whether it is a human *person*.' The question is not: 'When does a member of the human species come into existence?' but rather 'When does a human person come into

91

existence?' The problem now is not a matter of biology or embryology. So what is the nature of this problem?

III. Two false theoretical frameworks: mechanistic Darwinism and Cartesian dualism

14. Most of the fundamental problems of life are concerned with general attitudes of mind, with outlooks, with overall frameworks or points of view, more than with matters of detail. So it is possible that a person's limited outlook may prevent him from appreciating the true significance of the embryological facts and so from understanding the kind of biological beings we are; it may also prevent him from seeing the kind of personal beings we are. Let me draw your attention to two of these outlooks or frameworks which act like 'mental spectacles' through which reality is viewed, and, in fact, distorted. They are deeply ingrained in our society and underlie current evaluations of the whole of living reality in general and of the human conceptus in particular. One of these frameworks is mechanistic Darwinism and the other is Cartesian dualism; they are closely related.[2]

15. *Mechanistic Darwinism* is a form of 'scientism'. It is an outlook shared by many scientists and non-scientists. In this outlook the living being is regarded ultimately as nothing more than a very high-quality machine. Strictly speaking there are no living beings, but only inanimate reality. The living being is ultimately a well-organised conglomeration of molecules or a mass of cells. Molecules constitute the ultimate ingredients of life, its essence. They pass from generation to generation in a continuous chain; thus, life has no specific beginning or end, but is a process: 'nature is only a self-perpetuating machine'. In this perspective, to call an entity unique is to say simply that it is a combinatorial reassortment of molecules; this is the case with any living conceptus, as it is also the case with any mature ovum and sperm. Thus, the potentialities of living beings do not radically differ in nature from those of non-living entities and artefacts. A scientist involved in IVF, Dr H. W. Jones, has stated the point thus:

It is sometimes said that the embryo, if not a human person is potentially a human person, and therefore should be treated as such. But, in this sense, so is the egg or the sperm. A chassis with four wheels attached to the beginning of the assembly line is potentially an automobile, but no one would buy it for such until it was developed into an object which could be driven away from the end of the line. At the beginning, it is only potentially an automobile, just as is the iron ore from the mountains.[3]

If the reality 'life' is ultimately denied, through being 'explained' by appeal to mechanistic laws, and if the living being is reduced to combinations, replications and syntheses of molecules, how can the human embryo be understood? If after all life is no more than chemistry, the questions of morality and philosophy are non-questions, and whatever the true questions are, molecular physics and chemistry will provide the answers to them. Science will finally tell us what realities the words 'life' and 'person' really refer to. There is no realm of reality beyond the realm of scientific observation and theory.

16. The biological and philosophical significance and implications of recognising biological entities as living beings, that is, as organic living wholes, must be appreciated (contrary to the mechanistic outlook) if the natures of the embryonic and adult stages of our lives are to be appreciated. Let me point out here, very briefly, what I mean by saying that all living beings are wholes. A living whole is not merely a conglomeration of parts or particles, but a unity of function, that is, a being constituting internally a unity of life. It is not possible to understand adequately, or even to describe adequately, the nature of a living being without recognising it as a whole. There is enough evidence to show that every living being comes into existence as a whole, begins to be *itself* as a whole, grows as a whole, sustains itself as a whole, tends (if damaged) to heal itself as a whole, dies as a whole. Any parts of the living being (be they molecules, cells or full organs) can be understood *as* parts only if they are constitutive of the unity of the whole, if they function for the whole and in virtue of the whole. For parts do not function of themselves independently of the whole; rather, it is the whole that causes them to

93

function. Once removed from the whole, parts cease to be parts, cease to have an identity as parts, and they soon die since they are 'dis-integrated' from the whole. They are, in a sense, 'for' the whole, and the whole determines their constitution, function and proportion. Living beings are not 'heaps' or conglomerations of particles which can be easily dismantled and assembled back together again. They are *living* beings precisely because they have a life of their own, a unity of their own, from the beginning of their generation to their inevitable corruption in organic death. (For further discussion of the idea of living beings as wholes, see Chapter Six below, paras. 16–22.)

17. That living beings are not considered living wholes by some scientists can be illustrated by some comments of Sir Andrew Huxley, President of the Royal Society and Nobel Prize winner in physiology. He considers that there is an ambiguity in the use of the term 'embryo'. He wrote in the *New Scientist*[4] (and note the terminology he uses):

> The ambiguity arises because the word 'embryo' is also used to denote the *whole of the collection of cells* formed by repeated division of the fertilised egg during the first two weeks or so, although only a few per cent of these cells are destined to become the embryo proper; by far the greater number of them will turn into extra-embryonic tissue and ultimately into the structures that are discarded as the afterbirth. Furthermore, it is indeterminate which particular cells will form the embryo proper.

> The embryo proper is first recognisable at about the 15th day after fertilisation when a specialised region of cells called the 'primitive streak' first appears. Before that stage, it cannot be said that a definitive embryo exists: *the product of conception is a structure* of which a small and undetermined part will – if development proceeds normally – form a 'primitive streak' and later an 'embryo' in the sense in which the word is generally understood, and later again a 'fetus'.

18. What does it mean to say that 'the product of conception' is 'a structure'? Why is it not a living being in its embryonic form? Is the being generated as a whole at the 15th day? Are not the 'afterbirth', i.e., placenta and membranes, much-needed organs (organic parts) of the whole being which it

develops for its sustenance at the appropriate time and in correct proportion, as other parts are? Can the word 'pre-embryo', coined to abolish the alleged 'ambiguity' mentioned by Sir Andrew Huxley, prevent the embryo from being the living being generated and growing as a whole during the previous 14 days when it was a 'pre-embryo'? 'Cosmetic semantics' cannot change the nature of reality.

19. The second theoretical framework is *Cartesian dualism*. There is an intimate connection between mechanism and Cartesian dualism. The mechanists see the living being as a material conglomerate of particles, a 'structure' of parts, organised, functioning, but after all a 'machine' produced by nature, which sooner or later man will be able to comprehend, dismantle and assemble back again, and (it is hoped) produce better models. Physics can account for this machine. There is no soul to it. The French philosopher Rene Descartes conceived the human body in mechanistic terms as well, as a machine, but for him the machine had a soul. Thus, for him, the human being was a composite of two distinct realities. This is the reason why his philosophy of soul has been represented by the phrase 'the ghost in the machine'; the 'ghost' is the soul, the real 'I', a rational thinking being, the 'machine' is the body. Descartes reached this conclusion by ascribing the attributes of 'bodily' life to the machine; yet my real 'I' was not that. What was it? Descartes says:

> At last I have discovered it – thought; this alone is inseparable from me . . . I am, then, in the strict sense, only a thing that thinks; that is, I am a mind, or intelligence, or intellect, or reason, . . . a thinking thing.[5]

20. Two features of Cartesianism are most relevant to our present concerns. First, human beings are really to be valued for their rationality, for the thinking 'I'. The human body, the 'machine', is of importance in so far as it serves the thinking 'I', but in itself it is no better or worse than any other body (any other animal) or machine, since it is merely a biological organism like any other. Secondly, for the Cartesian it is possible to conceive the two realities, body and soul, as existing apart from each other at some stage, as well as together; so it is

possible to have a living body (of human kind) with no soul in it yet, and it is possible to have a soul existing without any body being attached to it. The human person is a body into which is 'infused' a rational soul. These views are common in contemporary debate, whether overt or implicit in what is being said.

21. The following question is frequently asked:[6] 'At what point in the development of the human organism, or of the human being, does the spiritual soul enter the human body?' This is the kind of question that someone dominated by Cartesian habits of thought can entertain, and currently it is a view widely held that the transformation of an entity from a mere biological being of human kind into a human person (i.e., a being with a rational soul) must occur at some stage. The evangelical geneticist Professor R. J. Berry has stated:

> It is a false extrapolation to assume that 'life' from God which transforms a biological being into a spiritual one is automatically given to every fertilised egg.[7]

A Catholic theologian, Professor John Mahoney, states the matter thus in his book *Bioethics and Belief*:

> ... it may be possible to have a human being which has not yet received a human soul infused by God and is therefore not yet a human person.[8]

Berry calls the early human being only a 'biological being', and Mahoney also uses the term 'biological node'. What are the reasons, the indicators, which suggest that the embryonic human being is not a personal being, that it is not endowed with an immortal soul? Professor Mahoney summarises the opinion of many in this matter when he says:

> the possibility of twinning and recombination in every conceptus (whether it occurs spontaneously or not) argues against a biologically stable subject for such immediate animation.[9]

22. An editorial in the British journal *The Economist* presents a similar mode of thinking in a popular manner, as follows:

> The question 'when does life begin?' is unanswerable. The classical theological answer – 'at conception' – is regarded by scientists as no longer fitting the evidence as they define it. Both sperm and

egg are alive before they join at fertilisation. But can a fertilised egg be described as the start of an individual life, when it may split into two and become twins – or when two eggs may fuse and become one? Can it be said to be on its way to humanity until 10–15 days later when it implants in the wall of the womb – an entrance test for 'life' that more than 50% of fertilised eggs fail?[10]

Thus, the fundamental reasons given as to why we may doubt that the human conceptus is a human person are ultimately founded both on empirical facts and on philosophical and theological doctrines. The empirical facts, we are told, put the 'philosophical and theological doctrine of the human soul . . . in a thoroughly unsatisfactory state'.[11] In what follows I shall briefly consider some of the fundamental issues related to the relevant empirical facts mentioned, and then focus on the doctrine of the soul.

IV. The wholeness of the living being; twinning and recombination

23. The biological picture we are given of twinning and re-combination in public debate (as distinct from the picture presented in good biology books) is constructed out of what is seen through the mechanistic or dualistic 'mental spectacles' mentioned above. The general picture we are given of the early embryo is a mechanistic one. It is said that the embryo is a conglomeration of 'undifferentiated' cells. So the embryo in these early days can enter or be brought into subsequent cellular divisions and aggregations of various kinds, and when these divisions, combinations and aggregations can no longer be brought about, we have a 'stable individual' which is no longer capable of becoming two or more (by twinning) or of fusing or recombining with another living being and thus 'becoming other'. It is claimed that the embryo, at this stage, is not a stable individual because 'it' can turn into two or more embryos, or can fuse with another embryo, the two individuals becoming now one. Further, a human person is constituted by a rational soul and so must be one and the same individual organism (i.e., one organic being) *continuously*. If this were not the case the soul – which is indivisible

97

and immortal – would have to 'divide' when the organic individual becomes two, or fuse, be lost or 'migrate' when one individual organism combines with another and both become one. But as this is not possible for an immortal indivisible soul, there cannot be a soul in the 'unstable' organic being that the early embryo is.

24. Let me dwell for a moment on the distorted scientific picture which underlies these views.

First, the organic mechanisms (whether molecular or cellular) of natural monozygotic twinning are not yet fully known or understood. There is not yet empirical and fully conclusive evidence to form a clear picture of *how* monozygotic twinning naturally occurs organically, either in human beings or in other animals in which twinning is possible. (In some forms of lower animals, e.g., ascidians, annelids, molluscs, twinning is not possible at all; it cannot even be induced artifically by division of the early embryo.[12]) It would be salutary to recognise this lack of knowledge on our part, and the realistic consequences of this lack for fundamental personal moral decisions or decisions of public policy. Theories based on data which are as yet unknown can only be speculative; they cannot have any stronger force than that.

Secondly, the mechanisms of embryonic 'fusing' or recombination are not known either. Furthermore, in this case, it is not even established that they do occur naturally, either in the human or in other mammalian species. Fusing and recombination can be deliberately induced, by either chemicals or by separation of cells (just as much as twinning can). The formation of 'chimeric' (and hybrid) animals has been attained by adding some cells to one kind of embryo, already developing in its early stages, from another (or others) of the same or of different species.[13] It is crucially important to be aware, in detail, of the conditions in which these experiments are carried out, in order to understand adequately the stage of development of each cell in the embryo, and of the embryo as a whole. For only under certain conditions are divisions and aggregations of cells possible; not every state or stage of change in a cell permits those manipulations. This detailed knowledge enables one to recognise the fact that although the individual cells of an embryo may be assimilated, integrated, into another living embryo, nevertheless once the embryo is killed *it* can assimilate nothing, even if some of its remaining cells can.

Thirdly, the early embryonic being cannot be regarded as a biologically 'undifferentiated' being, either molecularly or cellularly or morphologically; each embryo is always of a particular species, it is a single entity individuated in every respect and genetically unique. Biologists present us with evidence that molecular differentiating activity (in the cells of the conceptus both in the nucleus – the genes – and in the plasma, and both intra-cellular and inter-cellular) is at work from its formation and that it is continuously leading to full differentiation.[14] Visible differentiation of cells only reflects the emerging differences in their protein and enzyme content; the code for all proteins is spelled out by genetic messages reaching the cytoplasm from the nucleus. This molecular interaction between nucleus and cytoplasm is species-specific in the conceptus and active from its very beginning. Organically the embryo 'knows where it is going'. The law of its organic finality is dynamically written within itself at every stage of its existence from the time when, at fertilisation, it is formed as a conceptus.

Fourthly, it is indeed a fact that the *cells* of very early embryos can be disaggregated, aggregated, recombined to form chimeric or hybrid embryos in laboratory conditions (the 'geep', a hybrid of sheep and goat produced in a Cambridge laboratory, is a good illustration). But what these facts make clear is the regulatory capacity and powers that early embryonic beings possess in order (i) to make themselves complete and well-functioning again when some substantial part of the organism has been removed or damaged, and (ii) to assimilate or integrate into their organic wholeness molecular, cellular or organ parts from other organisms. In other words powers of grafting, transplant, healing and regeneration are present in the early living embryonic being. The fact that every living being is generated as a whole and develops as a whole does not, of course, alter the fact that this wholeness can be interfered with. Although there is a considerable amount of manipulation which an embryo as a living unity can endure and still survive, yet there are also limits to its ability to survive as a whole being.

25. As regards the 'aggregation' and 'disaggregation' of embryos (known to happen only by means of manipulations carried out under laboratory conditions) the most important point that must be made is this: we do have sufficient empirical evidence to establish that from an organic point of view, a living being does not divide as a whole being, as the living unity that it is, without being destroyed. Organically, because living beings are wholes constituted by parts (cells, organs), they can be manipulated, they can literally be 'mixed up'; yet this mixing-up is not of living beings as wholes (or of whole living beings) but of their parts. Let me give an example. If one cell of a four-cell sheep embryo is removed from the remaining three and put in a new *zona pellucida*, and allowed to develop on its own, it may give rise to a whole new sheep, and so will the other original three cells. (Experiments of this nature are described, for example, by S. M. Willadsen and C. B. Fehily: see note 13.) The individual cell, once separated, is a fragment which was a part of the embryo but now becomes a new whole being itself. But *before* the separation, the cell was a genuine part of the embryo because it was functioning as a part in relation to the whole, constituting it and not acting independently of the whole. Thus because a part (a cell) of an embryonic being has the capacity to become a whole if separated from it, we say the cell is *totipotential*; this is the case, for example, in the two-cell and four-cell sheep embryo. Nevertheless, the cell is not a whole as long as it is playing its own function, as a part, within the whole embryo.

26. The overall picture concerning living beings as wholes, and the relevance of this picture to the debate over twinning and recombination, may be presented in the following four propositions:

P1. A living being is an organic whole; as such it can shed parts (cells) which can become part of other organisms (through powers of 'grafting' and 'transplantation').

P2. A living being can shed parts (cells) which can become a new living being, a new organic whole itself, either on their own or in combination with another cell or cells (through powers of sexual and asexual generation).

P3. A living being can be deprived of, or damaged in, substantial organic parts (cells) and yet internally regulate the deficiency and continue to live and develop as a well-functioning whole (through powers of regulation, regeneration and healing).

The powers of the living being, as expressed in P1, P2 and P3, are not powers of division and fusion as they are often interpreted to be. Thus it may be claimed in addition that

P4. A living being, as a living whole, neither divides nor fuses with another whole being, as a whole being, although some of its parts (cells) can do so.

27. There can be *fragmentation* of living beings giving rise to asexual generation, but there is no 'fusion' and 'splitting' of living beings as total wholes. So, as there is no fusion and division of beings as wholes, the question of *organically* 'unstable' embryos does not arise; 'stable' individuality remains always a feature of every living being considered as a whole, even under conditions (whether natural or artificially-produced) which manifest the powers expressed in P1, P2 and P3 above. Every living being is a specifically and uniquely differentiated individual; that is, it is organically individuated from its generation to its death. *The early embryo, as a living whole, is an individual stable organism.* It is clear, then, that the recognition and understanding of the organic constitution of the living being in this manner does not bring into question the classical philosophical and theological doctrine of the soul. In other words, from a biological and philosophical understanding of living beings as wholes, it appears that 'the possibility of twinning and recombination in every conceptus (whether it occurs spontaneously or not) does not argue against a biologically stable subject for immediate animation'. (See above, paragraphs 20 and 21.) This topic of 'animation' is what I now propose to consider.

V. Philosophy and the truths of Christian faith

28. Let me first focus on the truths of Christian faith. Philosophical doctrines are not truths of revelation. Christian doctrines are not founded upon philosophical doctrines and do not

depend upon the latter for their truth. They are ultimately founded on the authority of God revealing. St Paul, in his attempt to form the Christian mind of the Corinthians, writes to them: 'in my speeches . . . there were none of the arguments that belong to philosophy . . . I did this so that your faith should not depend on human philosophy but on the power of God' (1 Corinthians, 2: 5). For this reason the task of the theologian rests on the following foundation:

> . . . that, accepting the truth of Catholic faith present in the living Church of which one is a member, one seeks a better understanding of this truth in which one already lives.[15]

Thus,

> theology neither calls into question the truth of faith nor attempts to prove it. There is no superior standard by which to criticize or establish the word of God.[16]

29. It is important for the Christian to recognise that truths of faith are living truths and attitudes held in the Christian community before they are ever formulated in principles and explained in doctrines. The divinity of Christ, on which Christianity is founded and without which it could not exist as Christianity, is a clear example of this. It was a reality first lived, shared and recognised by the community of Christians before it was challenged, distorted and threatened in its integrity. This challenge had to be met: explicit doctrinal formulations became necessary, and they did emerge in the life of the Church.

30. In the tradition of the Christian Church, respect for human life from conception has been a constant living truth and attitude since the Church's early days. This fact is well documented in recent historical studies. The principle of absolute respect for human life is already formulated in the *Didache*, one of the earliest Christian documents, dating from the beginning of the second century.[17] The same principle is constantly reiterated by the Fathers,[18] and, as a recent and authoritative pronouncement of the Church's teaching authority makes clear, 'it has never changed and it is unchangeable'.[19] It is a principle which the Catholic bishops of today, in agreement with their fellow bishops of the past, proclaim unanimously in

their pastoral and teaching work. A recent historical study of the Roman Catholic perspective on the destruction of unborn life makes this point:

> Early condemnations of abortion were generally associated with similar condemnations of infanticide, an indication that in the minds of the early Christians the two were closely related. The condemnation of abortion did not depend on and was not limited in any way by theories regarding the time of fetal animation. Even during the many centuries when Church penal and penitential practice was based on the theory of delayed animation, the condemnation of abortion was never affected by it. Whatever one would want to hold about the time of animation or when the fetus became a human being in the strict sense of the term, abortion from the time of conception was considered wrong, and the time of animation was never looked on as a moral dividing line between permissible and immoral abortion. As long as what was aborted was destined to be a human being, it made no difference whether the abortion was induced before or after it became so. The final result was the same: a child was not born.[20]

31. The principle of respect for human life from conception is, therefore, one of those principles which is constitutive of a Christian way of life. This way of life can be characterised, following J. H. Newman,[21] as foundational, enduring, unchangeable, general – yet immediately ethical and practical – dependent on conscience and embodying the essentials of an idea, namely, the 'vision' of human conception and of the human being from 'God's perspective'. To abandon so fundamental a principle is to move in the direction of dissolving a body of doctrine meant to protect and manifest a way of life in which each human being, while a corporeal being of flesh and bones, is also seen as God's creation, endowed with eternal life and an eternal destiny.

32. In this context, I see the task of any Christian thinker as an attempt to reach a better understanding of the truths of faith concerning the kinds of beings we are, and to draw out the implications of these truths for our actual behaviour. To abandon these living truths is to abandon the task itself. I consider the following to be truths of faith:

(i) Each human being is created by God as a unique personal being 'in his image'.

(ii) Each human being is called to share with God, and with others, God's eternal life and friendship.

(iii) We are to respect each other unconditionally as children of God, and we are never to destroy, harm or exploit any human being from conception until death.

(iv) The Word of God, Jesus Christ, became flesh, assumed our human bodily nature by his Incarnation, and became 'one of us' from his conception.

33. These truths are totally independent of scientific or philosophical doctrines. Therefore the teaching office of the Church cannot be asked for 'convincing' explanations of a philosophical or scientific nature in order to make the truths of faith acceptable or intelligible. These truths stand on their own grounds. The truth that the human conceptus is to be respected unconditionally from its generation is (as the Vatican's *Declaration on Procured Abortion* (1974, para. 13) states) 'perfectly independent of the discussions on the moment of animation'. This is so because the doctrine of 'ensoulment' or 'animation' is a *philosophical* doctrine. I shall briefly consider this doctrine now.

34. If one is to understand the whole question of animation, it is crucial that one should have an adequate appreciation of the philosophical conception of the soul, as it is discussed and explained first by Aristotle and then by subsequent philosophers, in particular by St Thomas Aquinas. Also, it is necessary to realise that the reality which corresponds to the concept of the soul can be described today with the additional help of modern explanatory language which derives from our new appreciation of various biological facts and of other aspects of the nature of the human person. I cannot, on this occasion, present the doctrinal development that has taken place, but there are certain things that can be said to put the current debate in some perspective.

First (as mentioned above) we must pay attention to the true description of the facts of early embryonic life. I believe that when these facts are adequately stated, the problems to which the early life of the human embryo is said to give rise disappear.

Secondly, it is important to recognise that neither Aristotle nor Aquinas maintained that there could be a living being of human kind, or a living being of human nature, a human being, which was not also a *homo*, 'one of us' – or, as we say today, a human person. They would have refused to accommodate the current distinction between 'human being' and 'human person', considered as referring to two different realities, one conceived as *biologically* human and the other as *rationally* human; these realities, according to some current authors, need not be present at the same time in one and the same thing. For Aquinas if a being is human, a member of the human species, that being is inseparably both physically (biologically) and rationally human. There cannot be a being who is bodily (physically) human and not rationally human, or vice versa. To be a bodily being of human kind is the necessary and sufficient condition for being a *homo* and so for possessing human nature, which is, of course, rational nature. Thus, to have a human body is to have a rational nature (a nature constituted by a rational soul, the soul being the form of the body). The corresponding situation applies in the case of animals: to have a canine body is to be a dog, and so to have a canine nature.

35. The general opinion among scholars concerning Aquinas's views on human and animal generation is summed up by one of these scholars in the following words:

> Aquinas, following Aristotle, held that in human generation [as in animal generation] two preliminary substantial forms – one by which the embryo is alive [vegetative soul], succeeded by one by which it is alive and has sensation [sensitive soul] – are present before animation by the rational soul (*ST* 1a, 76, 3, ad 3; 118, 2, ad 2), the sole substantial soul for man, according to 1a, 76, 4 . . .

> This opinion is based on two considerations: The philosophical principle that since form and matter are proportioned, there must be an appropriate disposition in matter to sustain the form; and the judgment, based on Aristotelian biology, that there is not sufficient organisation in matter at the time of human conception to sustain a rational soul. Contemporary Thomists generally accept the philosophical principle, not St Thomas's biological information. Modern genetics point to the complex organisation

present at the moment of conception, and so to a basis for affirming the temporal coincidence of conception and human animation.[22]

36. Let me consider further a philosophical aspect of the relationship between matter and form. For Aquinas, as well as for Aristotle, it was not possible to maintain that an animal was bodily and of a specific kind and yet did not possess the nature (form, soul) of that kind. When a living body (i.e., an animal) was so constituted as to be materially identifiable as a being of a particular kind, it was affirmed that that body was necessarily 'informed' with the soul (the substantial form) of that kind. In other words, these philosophers would have said that there could not be an animal, say a horse, whose bodily constitution was equine without the animal's *being* a horse. To be materially of a particular kind amounted to being a being of that kind. For this reason, these philosophers could not maintain that there could be an animal which was physically identifiable as human while not being a *homo*, a man, that is, a being possessing human nature and so 'in-formed' by a rational soul. This is so because of the inseparability of matter and form. Matter could only be identified as of a particular kind in virtue of its form; it is form which makes a being be what it is.

37. Aquinas repeatedly expresses this thought in propositions like the following:

. . . the soul is the actualisation of a body, meaning that due to the soul it is a body, and is organic, and has the power to live (. . . *anima est actus corporis etc., quia per animam et est corpus et est organicum et est potentia vitam habens.*) (*ST* 1a, 76, 4, ad 1.)

Human flesh is not human before it has the rational soul. (. . . *non prius est caro humana quam habeat animam rationalem.*) (*ST* 3a, 6, 4.)

Human flesh receives its being through the rational soul. (. . . *caro humana sortitur esse per animam.*) (*ST* 3a, 6, 4, ad 1.)

This is the insight which philosophically, is still valuable for us in our attempt to understand the nature of material living beings. Nevertheless, because Aristotle and Aquinas lacked biological information which is available to us today, neither of them could identify the natures of the different types of conceptus (either in man or in other animals such as the horse)

106

as we can today. They had no possible access to the organic (material) constitution of the different kinds of animal embryos, and were therefore unable to identify their differences. For this reason these philosophers thought that animal embryos were first *of non-specific kind*; any type of animal embryo was first an animal with a general animal nature but with no specific nature; therefore every embryo had to undergo a substantial change (a change of nature, a change of form, a change of soul) from an animal embryo in general to an embryo of a specific kind (human or equine). This view is untenable today, because we know that every animal embryo can be identified organically as possessing a specific nature, that is, as a member of a particular species right from its origin: we know that general natures do not exist concretely.

These ideas may be illustrated by some statements of Aquinas himself. He writes, for example, that

> the philosopher [Aristotle] says that the embryo is animal before it is a man. (*Philosophus dicit quod embryo est prius animal quam homo.*) (*ST* 1a, 76, 3; the reference is to the *De Generatione Animalium* II, 3, 736b2–5.)

– and it is clear that he shares Aristotle's opinion on this score. Aquinas also states:

> In animal generation the general animal nature is generated before the man or the horse. (. . . *in generatione animalis prius generatur animal quam homo vel equus.*) (*ST* 1a, 119, 2.)

> We must say that . . . since the coming into existence of a being involves the dissolution of another being, it must be held that, both in the case of men and of other animals, when a more perfect form supervenes this brings about the dissolution of the preceding one. However, it does so in such a way that the second form possesses whatever the first one does and something more into the bargain. And thus in man, as in the other animals, the final substantial form comes about through many comings-into-being and dissolutions. *'This is apparent in the case of animals brought into being by the process of putrefaction.* Therefore it must be said that the intellective soul is created by God at the completion of man's coming-into-being. This soul is at one and the same time both a sensitive and a nutritive life-principle, the preceding forms having been dissolved. (*Et ideo dicendum est quod cum generatio unius semper sit corruptio alterius, necesse est dicere quod tam in homine quam in*

animalibus aliis, quando perfectior forma advenit fit corruptio prioris; ita tamen quod sequens forma habet quidquid habebat prima, et adhuc amplius. Et sic per multas generationes et corruptiones pervenitur ad ultimam formam substantialem, tam in homine quam in aliis animalibus. Et hoc ad sensum apparet in animalibus ex putrefactione generatis. Sic igitur dicendum est quod anima intellectiva creatur a Deo in fine generationis humanae, quae simul est et sensitiva et nutritiva, corruptis formis praeexistentibus.) (*ST* 1a, 118, 2, ad 2; my emphasis.)

38. I should like to point out that these views of Aristotle and Aquinas concerning the different generations and corruptions involved in the formation of embryos were fraught with difficulties for them, and provoked criticisms from contemporaries and from philosophers in later times. And it was the paucity of the biological information available to them that led them to maintain that substantial changes (changes in which a living being either comes into existence or ceases to exist, changes involving generation and corruption, changes from one type of soul to another) could occur in the development of one and the same embryo. This was credible to Aristotle and Aquinas on the basis of what they took to be an unassailable scientific fact, namely, 'spontaneous' generation which required a substantial change, involved in the generation of living animals from dead putrefying matter, as the above passage indicates. We know today that spontaneous generation cannot take place.

39. A final point. It is to Aquinas's credit that he was able to conceive the possibility of there being an entity which would possess the complete nature of its progenitor from the very first moments of its formation as an embryo. But St Thomas judged the idea to be unacceptable (*hoc autem est inconveniens*, he says) given the biological facts as he took them to be:

> ... unless it was said perhaps that this dissolving process derived from all the parts and retained the nature of all the parts [of the progenitor]. Thus the semen would be, as it were, *a minute animal in existence* and the generation of animal from animal would simply come about by a process of division as, for example, mud is made up out of mud, and as occurs in the case of animals which keep living when cut in two. This view however is unacceptable. (... *Nisi forte quis dicat quod esset resolutum ab omnibus partibus*

*corporis, et quod retineat naturam omnium partium. Et sic semen esset quasi quoddam **parvum animal in actu;** et generatio animalis ex animali non esset nisi per divisionem, sicut lutum generatur ex luto, et sicut accidit in animalibus quae decisa vivunt. Hoc autem est inconveniens.*) (*ST* 1a, 119, 2; my emphasis.)[24]

40. In the light of the fundamental Aristotelian philosophical principle, shared by Aquinas, that 'what a thing becomes corresponds to what it first was' (*Finis rei respondet ejus principio, ST* 1a, 118, 3, 3), and in the light of our present biological information, we cannot avoid concluding that Aquinas *today* would have considered the human embryo from conception a *homo*, a being of human nature, a human bodily being endowed with a rational soul, 'one of us', a human person.

41. It is in and through our bodies that we are the specific kind of beings we are: our bodily constitution has the kind of personal humanity that all members of the human family share. The living human organism is the living human person. From conception to death every human being is a personal being, a being of human nature, in virtue of which his life and bodily integrity are at every stage to be respected.

42. I venture to suggest that the *major* problems of our time related to human generation are not 'intellectual', to be solved by intellectual and scholarly means (although these means are so important). Our problems, as human problems, have always been and remain primarily moral: 'a crisis of truth and responsibility in human relationships'. In a speech in the House of Lords the Anglican Bishop of Norwich quoted the following words of John Paul II. I should like to finish with them:

> The world has largely lost respect for human life from the moment of conception. The world is weak in upholding the indissoluble unity of marriage. It fails to support the stability and holiness of family life. There is a crisis of truth and responsibility in human relationships. And so I support with all my heart those who recognise and defend the law of God that governs human life. We must never forget that every person, from the moment of conception to the last breath, is a unique child of God and has a right to life. (*Hansard*, 31 October 1984.)

6

Death and the beginning of life

*I. The controversy concerning criteria for 'being dead' and for
'being alive'*

1. The viewpoint defended in the following passage by Peter
Singer and Deane Wells is a common one in current debate:

> The internationally recognised criterion for the permissibility of
> using vital parts of another human body is brain death. Total brain
> death, the complete absence of all brain functions, indicates that
> the heart, the kidneys and pancreas, and other organs may be
> removed for transplant purposes. If the medical profession (and
> indeed the Churches) recognise a body's lack of a functional brain
> as sufficient ground for declaring that there is no living person
> existing in that body, and the body may therefore be used as a
> means to worthwhile ends, then why not use *the same criterion at the
> other end of existence*? We suggest that the embryo be regarded as a
> thing, rather than a person, until the point at which there is some
> brain function. Brain function could not occur before the end of
> the sixth week after conception; it may eventually be shown that it
> does not occur until quite some time after.[1] (my emphasis)

2. The question 'Why not use the same criterion for determining the beginning and the end of existence?' is the central
question in this paper. It indicates that our consideration of the
coming-into-existence (the beginning-to-live) of the human
being, and his or her going-out-of-existence (ceasing-to-live)
refer to the same kind of entity. Thus, the questions of what it
is for a human being to be dead and what it is for him or her to
be alive are inseparable from each other. For we know what it
must be for someone to be dead only if we know what it is for

110

him to be alive; to declare someone dead is precisely to recognise and declare that he has ceased to be alive. Currently, physicians accept that the presence of certain criteria of brain death permit a legitimate diagnosis and determination of death of the whole person. Obviously those criteria must be related to what counts as death for them, that is, to their conception of death, what they take death to be. Criteria which are unrelated to or detached from what they are supposed to be criteria of – the death of a patient – cannot be acceptable. It follows that a commitment to certain criteria for determing death is also a commitment to a particular conception of death. By implication this same commitment must, then, involve a commitment to a conception of what it is for a patient to be alive – so that when he ceases to be alive he is then declared dead. No double standard can possibly apply in the two intrinsically-related situations: the life and death of one and the same human being.

3. A recent publication, *Death: Beyond Whole-Brain Criteria* (ed. R. Z. Zaner, 1988), resulting from a symposium held in the United States on the topic 'When are you dead?', presents the following point of view:

> At one stage of this debate, the President's Commission for the Study of Ethical Problems in Medicine and Biomedical and Behavioural Research recommended a uniform definition of death focused on the cessation of all brain functions, including those of the brain stem. Philosophical, ethical and practical issues provoked by individuals who have permanently lost consciousness, but whose brain stem still functions, demonstrate the impossibility of that recommendation, the contributors to this volume argue: their essays thus provide the basis for further critical examination of what it means to cease to be a person in the light of continual new developments in our biomedical understanding of the human brain. As it is now possible to sustain organic bodies which will never again house a conscious person, the contributors to this volume urge that it is necessary to reexamine what it means to be a person alive or dead in this world, and thus reexamine the basis for public policy.[2]

4. The concept of someone's being alive which is implied in the Singer–Zaner position – a position shared by many other

authors – is relative to a particular conception of the human person. For Singer and Zaner, the human person is to be distinguished from the human being, that is, from the living organic body: human personal existence is different from human bodily existence. For, as they put it, a living human body may 'never again house a conscious person'. A living human organism, that is, a body whose brain stem still functions, may nevertheless be damaged in such a way that consciousness is permanently lost, and as far as our understanding of the brain goes, it can never be recovered again. In this situation the living bodily being, according to the doctrine of this school, is not a human person any more. That one is a human being, a living bodily being of human species, does not necessarily imply that one is a person, 'a citizen' (to put it in more practical terms) entitled to the respect and to the natural and legal rights which pertain to persons. To be alive, according to Singer and Zaner, can only mean 'to be alive as a person' (in their sense of 'person'); hence to be dead equally means 'to be dead as a person' (in that same sense). The distinction made by these authors between 'the living body' and 'the living person' is based on an *a priori* determination of what is valuable in human existence, or what is 'essential to human existence'.[3] On this view, what is valuable in human beings is not their human bodily existence (let me call it their 'human nature') but their cognitive existence (their 'rational nature'), and for these authors human nature and rational nature are not the same thing. 'Rational nature' is absent if the capacity for ratiocination is absent because the brain is non-functional; and this may be due to the stage of embryonic development reached so far, or to a brain deficiency, disease or injury. In other words, the statement that someone is alive can be made truly if and only if that someone fulfils the necessary and sufficient conditions, established *a priori*, for an entity to have 'personal identity' and so to fall under the concept of a person, to count as a person and to be treated as one. Thus, 'being alive' and 'being dead' do not count as natural events which are universally discernible.

5. There is no need to stress that this particular conception of person (which in fact does not refer to beings of a general class

112

or species, of a 'natural kind' such as the human kind) would be prior to the criteria of death and life. The authors defending these views wish to bring it about that their concept of person, and the criteria for determining life and death which are bound up with this concept, are accepted in medical and legal contexts. So far this proposal has been widely rejected. What will be said in this paper will disclose some of the fundamental reasons for this rejection.

6. In what follows I intend to consider the criteria actually used in clinical practice, that is, in 'official medicine', for determining death, considered as brain death. This will enable to see the relationship that there is between, on the one hand, this concept of death and the criteria for determining it, and, on the other, the criteria determining the beginning of life. By contrast with the Singer–Zaner position, my exercise will show that the clinically accepted criteria for determining brain death offer good grounds for holding that human bodily existence (human nature) and human bodily death are the existence and death of *someone*, of a human subject. Hence neither the adult living human bodily being whose brain functioning is defective, nor the living human embryonic being, should be regarded as a thing that can be disposed of, but must be considered a human subject, a 'someone' to be treated with the respect due to the human subject. Let me advance here a formulation of the central contention of this chapter, which will be substantiated by the body of evidence to be provided. *The medical profession, which has the responsibility for officially declaring that someone is dead, is and has always been of the view that a patient is, without qualification, the living human bodily being, that is, 'the human living organism as a whole', and its practice has always been in accordance with this view. Furthermore, knowledge gained recently, which permits us to understand death as brain death, confirms this conviction and the corresponding medical practice.*

7. From the outset it must be stated that in spite of the common talk about brain death as 'the internationally recognised criterion' for permitting the use of vital organs for transplantation, strictly speaking, from a legal point of view, there is no international recognition as yet of the fact that

113

'brain death is death'. Further, there is no such thing as an internationally recognised criterion for determining that brain death has taken place. Medical standards also vary from country to country. In the USA a large majority of states (46 in 1988) have legal statutes recognising that brain death is death, but other states do not accept this view;[4] so a person might be considered dead in one state but not in another. In 1981 the President's Commission which studied these issues produced a report, *Defining Death*, which sought to reach a uniform determination of death. Similar attempts (legal and medical) have been made in European countries as well.[5] There are international efforts within the medical profession to come to an agreed non-arbitrary standard for the declaration of brain death as an event identifiable with death. Such a universal standard would indeed be desirable, for most of us would share Professor I. M. Kennedy's misgivings when he says that it would be 'in no way inspiring of confidence in one's doctor to learn that there are two types of death'.[6] There is no doubt that there should be a medical answer to the question. 'Is this patient dead?' – an answer 'based on medically defined, clearly formulated and well publicised criteria', as has been rightly demanded.[7]

8. Although I am aware that there is not as yet a universally adopted criterion for determining brain death (and hence that there is not yet any universal understanding and agreement as to what constitutes brain death), I need to base my own considerations here on a particular understanding of 'brain death'. There are three main views of what 'brain death' may mean. The first is the 'neocortical view of death',[8] according to which, when the higher brain functions, the neocortical functions, are irreversibly lost, the upper brain is dead and so the patient as a person is dead, even if the brain stem is still functioning. This is the Singer–Zaner view mentioned above. The second is represented by the US Uniform Determination of Death Act (UDDA), which states:

> An individual who has sustained either (i) irreversible cessation of circulatory and respiratory functions, or (ii) irreversible cessation of all functions of the entire brain, including the brain stem, is dead. A determination of death must be made in accordance with accepted medical standards.[9]

114

The third view is exemplified by the 'Memorandum on the Diagnosis of Death', adopted in the United Kingdom by Medical Royal Colleges and Faculties in 1979,[10] and also by the 'Memorandum on Brain Death' adopted in Ireland in 1988.[11] In these memoranda it is maintained that death has been established when all functions of the brain have permanently and irreversibly ceased. Recent medical developments have confirmed that the necessary and sufficient condition for the ending of all functions of the brain, that is, for whole-brain death, is the death of the brain stem.[12] In other words, if the brain stem is diagnosed as totally and truly dead, then the whole brain must be considered dead, and so the patient may be declared dead. Dr Christopher Pallis, neurologist at the Royal Postgraduate Medical School in London, who has greatly contributed to the understanding of brain-stem death, has stated:

> If the brain stem is dead, the brain as a whole cannot function, and if the brain has permanently lost the ability to function, the individual is dead.[13]

9. There has been controversy in British and Irish circles as to whether the tests used for the diagnosis of brain-stem death are fully adequate to establish that the brain stem is indeed irreversibly dead,[14] and whether the present identification of death as brain-stem death is adequate. The controversy still continues. But the fact of this controversy does not affect my central claim. For the British–Irish position and the American position are agreed on one point, namely, that *ultimately* the death of the whole brain means the death of the patient; the difference between the two positions is a matter of the different ways in which they understand the relation between death of the brain stem and death of the whole brain. I therefore assume in this discussion that 'brain death' is not to be defined as 'neocortical brain death' (or higher-brain death), that death does not ultimately mean 'the death of the brain', but rather 'the death of a human being, as determined by an examination of brain functioning' which establishes that the brain is dead.[15] I therefore disregard the controversy as to whether the process of determining that brain death has occurred is adequately

carried out by the medical means which are used at present in diagnosing brain-stem death. For convenience's sake, I shall refer to the view adopted here as the Anglo-American 'total brain death' conception (abbreviated TBD). The discussion which follows will be divided into three parts. In the first part I shall describe the fundamental aspects of the medical under-standing of TBD. Then I shall discuss some of the basic philosophical concepts on which this understanding rests. Finally, I shall draw conclusions which derive from such a position concerning the beginning of life of the human being, so that no double standards or criteria are applied for deter-mining the coming-into-existence and for the going-out-of-existence of one and the same being.

II. 'Brain Death' as the basic criterion for death: physiological facts

10. The following two theses are the most basic constitutive tenets of TBD, the Anglo-American position as regards brain death:

(a) Brain death is the death of the living human organism as a whole;
(b) The death of the living human organism as a whole is the death of the patient, the death of a human subject.

Both in the American and in the British context it has been emphasised that the absence of 'functions' in the brain must not be confused with the occurrence of

activity in cells or groups of cells . . . (metabolical, electrical, etc.) [which] is not manifested in some way that has significance for the organism as a whole. [16]

Dr Christopher Pallis has written:

The irreversible cessation of heart beat [blood circulation] and respiration implies *death* of the patient as a whole. It does not necessarily imply immediate death of every cell in the body . . .

The irreversible cessation of brain stem function implies death of the brain as a whole. It does not necessarily imply immediate death of every cell in the brain. [17]

Death . . . is the dissolution of the organism as a whole. [18]

116

The truth of statements (a) and (b) depends on certain physiological facts as well as on a key concept, that of the organism as a whole, which underlies the understanding of TBD. Unless that concept is truly applicable to the human organism, the view that the death of a patient's brain is the death of the patient himself would not be justified.

The medical profession has always established death on physiological grounds, in basically the same manner as we all do in diagnosing the deaths of our pet animals. The traditional criteria for determining death, which for the majority of people is readily diagnosed at the bedside, are the cessation of the functioning of heart and lung, that is, cessation of blood circulation and of spontaneous breathing, together with the other known signs which accompany the cessation of these functions. This is so because we take circulatory and respiratory functions to be necessary for human life. Let me call this the traditional view of what the diagnosis of death consists in. In recent decades, certain machines (in particular the medical respirator) have been developed to assist or take over these functions of respiration and blood circulation by causing oxygen to flow in to the lungs of the patient and by pumping blood through his body. In this context a question arises: Does the presence of ventilation and cardiac action induced by a machine always indicate the presence of a living human being? Does the existence of these functions always indicate that the patient is alive? The answer is in the negative, because the origin of these functions may be totally artificial, i.e., machine-produced, so that they are not the result of any brain operations in the human subject. (I assume here that this is what actually occurs when clinicians tell us that a human corpse is ventilated and that the heart beats and blood flows). Naturally, if there is persistent spontaneous cardiopulmonary activity in (e.g.) a comatose patient, that is sufficient for concluding that a human life remains, that the patient is still alive. (Issues concerning the correct mode of medical treatment and care for patients in a coma or in a vegetative state should not be confused with issues concerning the determination of death.) It is important to note that a patient may be in a vegetative state (that is, maintaining spontaneous breathing but with no self-consciousness) for long periods of time:

117

Karen Quinlan, for example, was in that state for over ten years. As regards the vegetative state, Dr Pallis claims that 'no authoritative medical or legal body has, to my knowledge, ever defined the vegetative state as death', and that 'no culture has ever considered patients in the vegetative state as dead, or as suitable subjects for organ donation'.[19] As far as clinical practice and clinical judgement are concerned, a spontaneously breathing human being is a living person, a patient. Modern physiological studies have made it clear that if breathing persists the brain is not dead, because the brain stem is alive. In the past, and for the majority of people today, including doctors, a 'breathing human body' is a living human being, a living person. (It is generally *philosophers* who hold to the neocortical definition of death, and those who follow their views, who disagree with this position.)

11. More accurate knowledge of physiology has enabled us to establish also that when the brain has ceased to function, the unity and integration of vital functions have irreversibly broken down. It can then be said that there is no living organism, no unified life, no living human being. We are told that it is now possible to maintain artificially a group of bodily subsystems in a disintegrated, non-unified dead body.[20] However, this does not bring the traditional view of death, understood as the cessation of cardiopulmonary functions, into opposition with the total-brain-death view.[21] For the latter view recognises that the vital organs – heart, lungs and brain – have a special significance in maintaining the integrated, unified functioning of the organism as a whole. Other organs like the kidneys or the skin do not have this significance. In the former set of organs the 'interrelationship is very close and the irreversible cessation of any one very quickly stops the other two'.[22] It is known that if the brain is deprived of blood flow (and so of oxygenation) for 10 to 15 minutes it will completely cease to function, including the brain stem. Even if circulation is only partially impaired, loss of function of some of the brain neurons will occur.

12. Advances in medical knowledge, accompanied by current techniques, have enabled us to realise more clearly than ever

before that human death is, and has always been, brain death. This is a real development in our understanding of the physiological nature of death which permits us to establish proper criteria for determining and declaring death. The clinical as well as the common-sense understanding of death as *death of the living being*, that is, *death of the human organism as a whole*, is seen to be a common element in both the traditional and the more recent approach to thinking about death. It is clear that biological criteria, that is, bodily organic criteria, have traditionally been ultimately decisive for determining death. Seen in this light, the TBD position does not contradict, but rather complements, develops and further clarifies the traditional position as regards the determination of death for a human individual. Both positions maintain that the death of the patient is the death of his living organism: it is his organic death. Hence to be a living human organism is the necessary and sufficient condition for being a living patient, a living human being, a human subject.

13. We may ask the question: What or who is it that is declared dead when a human brain is said to be dead? In the light of what has been said, the answer obviously is that what is dead is, in general terms, 'the living being', and in human terms, 'the living human organism', which we may also take to mean 'a patient', 'a human subject'. When death is declared, the living organism is said to have ceased to be alive (as an 'independent biological unit', to use Dr Pallis's term). Here the view of the medical profession is in line with that of ordinary common sense, because if the human organism is found to be dead, what is really dead is the patient, the human subject. This is what the written death certificate informs us about. This fact is something which may appear too obvious to be worth mentioning, and yet it may not be sufficiently acknowledged that the patient in medical practice is rightly taken to be identical with his living organism. In other words, the death of the patient, for all legal, medical, familial and other human purposes, is his organic death, his biological death. It is clear, then, that the criteria related to such a concept of death as organic death must be organic criteria, physical criteria. According to current clinical thinking and practice, these are the

119

criteria which guide and are used in the implementation of appropriate clinical tests which show that the brain is dead.

14. When we talk about the death of a patient, we cannot but talk of the patient *as a whole*. Every doctor knows (as we all do) that when the living organism of the patient dies it is the patient himself who dies; he therefore recognises a fundamental truth concerning the human condition, namely that every human being is a bodily being, an organic being. If the organic being dies the human subject dies. This view does not imply that a patient is nothing but his organic make-up, but it certainly does imply that the patient *is* indeed his organism. And this is what is fundamental for the determination of his death. The medical profession has not, does not and should not treat patients as other than bodily beings; they are of a very specific nature, a human and rational nature, but human rational beings are bodily beings after all.

15. The fact that death is organic death, bodily death, is of universal significance: it applies, that is, to every human being. Every human being, of every culture and nation, can appreciate this mode of understanding death. Our bodily condition is a universal human feature which we all share. We all share *humanity*. If doctors are to act as doctors, in whatever part of the globe they may exercise their skill, they have to be concerned with human subjects as bodily beings. Their understanding of what it is to be dead or to be alive cannot vary according to the modes of thought fashionable in a particular society which may be unduly influenced by a particular school of thought involving some restricted account of what counts as a person. If patients were to be forced to recognise radically different concepts of death, they would have to accept the existence of at least two types of death, and perhaps even more. (Obviously, if there is more than one way of being alive, there must be more than one way of being dead.) The universal significance of death demands that the same term 'death' should refer to the same physical conditions. Death is a natural event which we are called upon to recognise, both in human beings and in other animals; it cannot be described in terms which ignore its natural reality.

III. Philosophical considerations:
(i) 'The organism as a whole'

16. When we talk about the human being, and about his death, we typically use such terms as 'living organism', 'an individual', 'an independent biological unit', 'the organism as a whole', etc. We could also, of course, use those expressions if we were talking about (say) a dog. This is so because these modes of expression involve a commitment to a fundamental biological truth concerning living beings in general, namely, that they are living organisms, and that living organisms are living wholes, units of life, and not mere conglomerations of parts. Their true identity is constituted, and must be understood, as the existence of a living organic totality, a living being that is a living whole. We could not accept either the traditional or the brain-death criterion of death as organic death without also accepting that the living being is a living organic whole. We enter now into the consideration of basic philosophical concepts which are presupposed in every understanding of what it is to be alive or dead. The truth about the wholeness of living beings is a non-scientific truth which nevertheless grounds the physiological (scientific) understanding of the nature of living beings. This concept of organic wholeness or of the organism as a whole is central to the TBD understanding of brain death as death.

17. The idea of wholeness could be understood in two different ways;[23] let me call them the quantitative and the qualitative modes of understanding. Death could be regarded either as the dissolution of *the whole organism*, or alternatively, as the dissolution of *the organism considered as a whole*. The first way of viewing death is the quantitative conception, and it involves identifying death with the dissolution of all the individual parts of the body – that is, of all the cells of the organism. Clearly this is not the criterion actually used for the declaration that someone is dead: a decapitated person, for example, is considered to be dead as soon as his head has been severed, even if the heart continues beating for a short time. It is not necessary that all the cells of an organism be dead for the organism itself – the organism as a whole – to be dead. What *is*

required for death is that the functional unity of the organism be destroyed. In any case, it could happen that many of the cells of an organism, and even some of its organs, would be dead while the organism itself, as a whole, remained alive. The term 'wholeness', in the sense being employed here, the qualitative sense, refers to the unity and integration of the organism, to its overall oneness of function, and not to the working of each individual cell and cell part.

18. We could not claim that an organism dies as a whole if it were not, before death, a single living being. It is therefore of great importance to appreciate the biological and philosophical implications of regarding living organic beings as organic wholes. The living organism manifests itself as a single whole by its unified organic constitution (its oneness of bodily form) and by its powers (its unified activity). The living organism is self-growing, self-organising, self-preserving, self-fulfilling, self-healing. We observe living organisms coming into being as living wholes and moving and functioning as wholes; we see that they grow and develop as wholes, relate to other living beings as wholes and eventually die as wholes. They are organic wholes endowed with the powers of self-movement and self-development. Admittedly, their bodies are constituted by parts which are heterogeneous; but the different parts of the whole being (cells and organs) develop in harmony and proportion with each other, and they manifest at every stage the unified organic activity of the whole.

19. The unity and power of the whole determines, and is prior to, the form and functioning of the parts. The whole produces all its parts for self-maintenance at every stage of its existence, tending towards its own maturity. The whole has priority over the parts. This is what constitutes the difference between the order of living organic wholes and the order of non-living, inorganic ones. As Auguste Comte says, it is 'the passage from an order in which parts precondition the whole to an order in which the whole shapes the parts, and, in a sense, precedes them'.[24] The parts of a living being, then, are there in view of the whole. The activity and constitution of the parts can be understood only in terms of the whole. An analogy with

machines may help us to appreciate this point better. The parts of which machines are composed are quite different from those of which living organisms are composed: machine parts are homogeneous in structure, and machines cannot substitute one part for another in case of failure, cannot regenerate or heal themselves and do not produce the energy that moves them. These differences between living organisms and machines are manifestations of the radical difference in kind between them as regards their wholeness. The machine is constructed, organised, assembled, from parts to whole. The living organism forms itself as a whole being; it moves and organises itself towards a state in which it is a mature specimen of its kind. In the living being the whole which is coming into being itself governs the formation of the parts. The living being is the dynamic law of its own development; the machine is not.

20. Clearly, if the order and organisation of the organic being is changed and undermined in a serious fashion, the being itself will cease to exist. None of the fundamental parts of the living being, the vital organs – brain, heart, lungs, kidneys, liver, etc. – is a biologically independent unit, capable of sustaining itself as a unit. Rather, it is the organism as a whole which is such a unit. Further, when the organism as a whole dies because one of its vital organs is destroyed, what is destroyed is precisely that fundamental unity and organisation of the being without which it cannot be itself, cannot exist.

21. Because the wholeness of the organism is not reducible to any of its parts, none of the parts can be given the status of the whole. It would be a mistake to regard any single organ, such as the brain, as somehow constituting the organism itself, of causing it to exist as a whole. If the whole is alive, it is already there with its own particular nature and powers; neither the presence nor the absence of one of its parts can account for the kind of unity which the whole is. Rather, the nature of the whole itself has primacy over the parts, as Comte pointed out in the passage quoted above. The whole organism comes to develop the specific parts that are appropriate to it precisely because of the kind of whole that it is.

123

22. Let me sum up the basic ideas developed here, concerning the organism as a whole, in the following seven propositions:

(i) the human organism (the human bodily being) is a living whole.

(ii) The organism as a whole is 'an independent biological unit', that is, a living organic individual.

(iii) The organism as a whole, the living unit (individual) that it is, is not the quantitative aggregation or the sum total of its parts, but is qualitatively distinct from that quantitative sum total.

(iv) This living unit or whole is not caused to exist by, nor is it constituted by, any one of its parts considered singly.

(v) The whole is not reducible to any of its parts.

(vi) The death of the whole may be caused by the destruction of one of its parts because the dissolution of a unified order could come about through the failure of that one organ (or part), leading to a substantial alteration of unity and of the organisation of the individual being.

(vii) The whole has primacy over the parts, for it determines their development, form, appearance and harmonious function both in space and in time. The whole determines the parts.

The fact that organisms are living wholes makes it reasonable to claim – given our present knowledge of the workings of the human organism – that anyone who has suffered brain death has suffered the loss of brain function, and therefore that death of the whole organism has occurred: the person himself has died. For centuries the fact that death of the brain and death of the whole organism were identical was intuitively obvious; it was an assumption which underlay such practices as decapitation and judicial hanging.

(ii) Death: an irreversible state

23. The following statements are sometimes made by people trying to describe what death really amounts to: 'Death is a state'; 'Death is a natural event'; 'Death is a process'. Which of these statements is true? Or are they all true? Are the statements compatible with one another? The description of death as a state seems to be justified, given that (as we have seen) the death of a living being is to be identified as the dissolution of the organism as a whole, that is, as the ending of the organic unity or wholeness of the living body. It is a true description in

124

so far as it implies that the death of a living being has already been identified in the dissolution of the organism as a whole – that is, when the organic unity or wholeness of the living body is acknowledged to have ended. The central idea behind the brain death criterion is that *there are empirical tests by means of which the brain can be declared dead and the whole organic body therefore declared to have lost its unity or wholeness.* While the process of dying is still going on, the organism is not yet dead, and it would be wrong to declare it to be so. This reveals that although dying is a process, death itself is not. When we want to determine that death has occurred, we have to ascertain whether the end of the process has yet taken place, and to do this we must have criteria for asserting that it has. Thus, when one determines that death has taken place, it is the end of the process of dying as well as the criteria used to detect that end which matter. The significance of the concept of brain death is precisely that it makes clear that there are relatively simple and non-arbitrary methods, usable by the bedside, by which it can be shown that the end of the process of dying has taken place. Death, then, is that state which is reached when the process of dying has come to an end. In this respect death can also be aptly described as an event, a natural event – that is, as an occurrence identifiable by certain criteria at a particular point in time (ordinary clock time). The question 'At what time did he die?' makes perfectly good sense, as does an answer such as 'At ten past six in the evening'.

24. Death occurs as an event both when it takes the form of a simultaneous destruction of every one of the cells of an organism (as when someone falls into a blast furnace at 1,000°C), and also when there is a gradual dissolution of the organism as a whole, that is, as a functioning unit. In both cases there has to be a point in time at which the dissolution (whether it occurs in the first or the second of the ways mentioned here), as the end of the process, can be seen to have occurred. Of course, it may be impossible, in practice, to identify the earliest point in time at which someone can be declared to be dead; the doctor has to carry out his tests and be completely satisfied that the end of the process has occurred. In this sense it is true to say that we are dead when the doctor says we are dead. But the doctor

125

makes this judgement on grounds which are not arbitrary; and the crucial problem here is to specify these non-arbitrary grounds for a judgement that death has occurred. Because dying takes time, it is a process, and it is of crucial importance for the doctor who declares death to take into consideration the necessity of *waiting*: it is ultimately by waiting, after having ascertained the known signs of dying and death, that the certainty of death is absolutely established for everyone concerned.

25. Strictly speaking, death is not a process as dying is.[25] A process is, by its very nature, extended over time. If death were a process, a declaration of death would have to be made during the time that the process was occurring; but then there would be no way of distinguishing between the process of dying and the process of death itself. As a consequence, the distinction between the three conditions of living, of dying and of being dead could not be made. This shows clearly that one must identify with certainty a definite dissolution of the living organism as a whole if one is to declare, on non-arbitrary grounds, that a patient is dead. The significance of the brain-death criterion is precisely that it shows that a non-arbitrary line can be drawn between dying and death: it shows that the end of the living process of the organism is clinically (empirically) determinable and that the organism is truly dead at a particular point when it is judged that the process has ended.

26. Irreversibility is another important aspect of death. That death is irreversible follows from the fact that the human organism is a living whole, and as such cannot be dismantled and reassembled as a machine can. We all realise that when the living unity of a human being has truly broken down, that unity can never again be recovered. If corpses were at any time liable to come to life again, we would not have criteria for considering the dead as really dead! Our understanding of living beings is such that their death is final, and this finality is irreversible, as the actual decomposition of the corpse manifests. So we may ask: What does the state of being dead consist in? The usual answer has been: 'It consists in the death of the

organism as a whole'. And when and how does the wholeness of the organism break down? According to the brain-death criterion, this happens when there is an irreversible loss of brain function. The next question which arises is: 'When does the loss of brain function occur, and how is it known?' Here physiology has to give us the answer.

(iii) The irreversible loss of function and capacity

27. The notions of function and capacity are not clearly differentiated in discussions of brain death. This is not surprising, since 'to function' and 'to possess a function' may be taken to mean 'to have a power or capacity for a particular activity'. We regard an activity as an exercise of a capacity or a power. Capacity and activity (or exercise of a capacity) are to be distinguished; they are not reducible to each other, although the latter depends on the former. The human mind has the capacity for thought; thinking is the activity corresponding to that capacity, its actual exercise. The human mind is more than a capacity for thought or consciousness; it could be aptly called a capacity for capacities.[26] To possess a mind is to possess the capacity to acquire other capacities, e.g., to learn how to walk and eat, to learn to speak, to learn a foreign language, to learn to drive or to play the piano. We may have all these capacities and not be able to exercise them for one reason or another. Naturally reasons may vary: I may not be able to play the piano because I am under an attack of panic which has paralysed me, because my hand has been hurt in an accident, because I have no piano. This example shows that we must make a further distinction between a *capacity*, its *exercise* and its *vehicle*.

28. A patient under total anaesthesia is in a state in which he is not capable of walking, feeling pain, being self-conscious, etc.; this state is caused, as a result of the anaesthesia, by the physiological changes affecting the organs which are the necessary bodily vehicles for these capacities to be exercised. Clearly the impossibility of exercising these capacities under anaesthesia cannot be taken as the loss of the capacities themselves, but should rather be understood as a temporary

127

'obstruction' of some of those vehicles by means of which the capacities can be actualised and exercised. If the vehicles were permanently damaged or destroyed the capacity would no longer be exercised, as (e.g.) in the case of a brilliant pianist who loses the movement of his hands. The exercise of a capacity and its vehicle are inseparable, so that if the vehicle is lost the possible exercise of the capacity is lost as well. As Anthony Kenny has argued,[27] a power, understood as a capacity, cannot be reduced either to its vehicle or to its exercise. Nevertheless this form of reductionism prevails among some scientists and philosophers when they identify the mind (which for them is the same thing as the person) with the *exercise* of consciousness. Others identify the mind with its vehicle, the brain, for they maintain that the mind is the brain.

29. It is necessary for our human way of describing ourselves that we have a term such as 'mind' which stands for those capacities of intelligence proper to our species. Yet the powers that a living being possesses (powers of generation, movement, growth, sight, etc.) are capacities of that being itself as an organic unified living whole, and are exercised through its organs. But it is not the organs that generate, move, see, etc., but rather the being itself. Obviously, if there is no organism there are no capacities, no powers. But if an organism is present then the capacities or powers which belong to its nature are also present, despite the many organic limitations, deficiencies or injuries it may have at present or may come to have in the future. Because powers have particular organs as their vehicles, destruction of or damage to some parts of my organism may deprive me of the means of exercising those powers. It is a fact about the human organism (and about other animal organisms) that when the whole brain is irreparably damaged or destroyed and therefore ceases to function, the organism can no longer maintain and exercise its unifying power of being alive as a whole, as a unit. Thus, the brain is one of the essential vehicles by which the living unity of the organism is maintained; the loss of this organ is the loss of that unity, the loss of the life of the organism. To be alive is to act and operate in a unified way. What is lost, then, when the

128

brain is irreparably damaged or destroyed is the constantly-active power of *being one*, of being in existence as such-and-such a kind of being; what is lost is the power of life itself. Losses of other organs of the human body may not amount to the total and irreversible loss which precludes the organism as a whole from living; the loss of the brain, however, does. This is a matter of physiology, of the way we are made, and it applies just as much to human beings as it does to the other animals.

(iv) A definition of death

30. Various definitions of death may be advanced. Death, like our personal being, or subjectivity, or sexuality, or our coming into being, escapes a fully satisfactory definition. Nevertheless there are definitions and descriptions which succeed in laying bare the essential features of these realities. The reality of death, from a medical point of view, has been defined by Dr Pallis in these terms:

> Death is a state in which there is irreversible loss of capacity for consciousness combined with the irreversible loss of the capacity to breathe (and hence to maintain a heart beat). Alone neither would be sufficient. Both are essentially brain stem functions (predominantly represented, incidentally, at different ends of the brain stem).[28]

This definition of death has been designed to fit in with the criteria given for brain-stem death, taking into consideration the importance of consciousness in human life. It is therefore a tentative definition. (It should be noted that Dr Pallis does not discuss the distinction between a capacity, its vehicle and its exercise.) The capacities irreversibly lost at death are said to be two: (a) spontaneous breathing, and (b) consciousness. Why is it that the definition specifies that these two capacities are to be lost? Why not one of them only? Why not others? The answers to these questions depend partly on certain results of modern technology and partly on human physiology, rather than on any philosophical principles or conclusions. The loss of spontaneous breathing does not always mean death. With the aid of a machine, and after appropriate tests, it can be determined whether the loss of breathing function is only temporary and could therefore be restored later, or whether it is a permanent and irrecoverable loss. If the loss is permanent, and if this loss is accompanied by loss of the capacity for consciousness, then death will have occurred: these two powers depend for their existence on the functioning of the brain stem, and since these powers 'reside' at opposite ends of the stem from each other, loss of both powers shows that the total stem is dead. (If this were not the case – if the stem were still partly alive – then Dr Pallis's definition of death would, of course, be inadequate.)

31. What all this reveals is, I believe, that it is a necessary condition for someone's being alive that his brain stem is alive; it is not, however, necessary that the neocortex, the vehicle which is required for the exercise of consciousness, is alive and functioning. The exercise of consciousness is irreversibly lost by a severely-damaged cortex even if the stem is well-functioning and not damaged. This is well illustrated by the fact that a child with hydroencephaly is a living child, even though he entirely lacks the capacities for ratiocination and reflexive self-consciousness:

> The child can breathe spontaneously, swallow, and grimace in response to painful stimuli. Its eyes are open. The heart can beat normally for months. No culture would declare that child dead. This emphasises the centrality we instinctively allocate to persisting brain stem function, even in the absence of what we could describe as cerebration.[29]

We have no way of ascertaining that capacities for consciousness and for breathing have been lost other than by testing to discover the physiological state of the brain stem. And if the brain stem is alive, the organism as a whole is still functioning, not dead. For this reason it is my contention that *if the brain stem is the crucial organ for determining death it is not because it contains the basic mechanisms for the exercise of the capacity for consciousness, and because consciousness is a 'philosophical' attribute relevant to determining life or death, but rather because if this organ is dead, the unity of the living organism is broken and hence all spontaneous vital powers and functions are destroyed along with it.*

A damaged, destroyed, dead brain stem detaches the higher brain from the rest of the organism, and as a result the unity of the living being is irreversibly lost. There is, then, no longer a living whole, a living bodily individual.

32. The concept of death expressed in the definition cited in paragraph 30 above is said to be

> a hybrid one, expressing both philosophical and physiological attributes . . . which corresponds perhaps to an intermediate stage of current concerns, seeking to maintain a footing on both types of ground.[30]

In my view, both physiological and 'philosophical' attributes will always be present in a human concept of death, given the kind of beings we are. Relying on current knowledge about the brain and the brain stem, I would defend a definition of death which includes both physiological and 'philosophical' characteristics which are recognised to be real in the human being (as in other animals). The definition is this:
Death is the dissolution of the organic unity that a being possesses as a living whole.

Of course, this definition does not capture the whole sense and reality of human death, since it could be applied to other animals; but it does express the fact that through death the human being ceases to exist as a human being. The 'dissolution of the organic unity of a being' is known to have occurred when the brain is found to be dead. This understanding of death is an organic, physiological one, although complemented and substantiated by philosophical insight into the nature and powers of the human organism as a living whole, a living organic being of human and rational nature. The human bodily nature that disintegrates at death could still be well expressed in the words 'the last breath'. When the brain dies, the head hangs down, breathing ceases, death ensues. Death as traditionally understood, on the one hand, and 'brain death', on the other, are and will always be one and the same.[31] There is only one kind of human death: organic death, death of the human organism as a whole, for such an organism is the human being, the human person.

IV. Death and conception compared

33. The end of human life we call death. The beginning of human life we call conception.[32] A question which arises here is whether the attributes which must be present if a living human organism is to be recognised as a human subject, a human being or a human person are the same attributes whether we are speaking of death or of conception. In what follows the criterion used for determining what counts as a living human subject who ceases to be alive and is therefore declared dead, when his or her brain is dead, will be applied in order to determine when that human subject began to be alive. In this application it will become clear that the set of 'conceptual commitments' in the nine propositions stated below represent those implied in the concept of death as total brain death, as discussed above. The other set of propositions represent the parallel commitments implied by the recognition of conception as the beginning of a human life. The legitimacy of the original question – 'Why not use the same criterion for determining the beginning and the end of human existence?' – is therefore made manifest.

34. I now state nine propositions concerning criteria for determining the end of life (death) and the beginning of life (conception).

P1 (Death): The living human subject, the dying patient, is the living human organism.

A human patient is a living human organism, a living whole, a member of the human species. To be such a kind of living human organism is the necessary and sufficient condition for one's being recognised as a living human subject, a human being, a human person.

P1 (Conception): The embryonic human being is the living human organism.

A human being in embryonic form is a living human organism, a living whole, a member of the human species. To be such a kind of living human being is the necessary and

132

sufficient condition for one's being recognised as a living human subject, a human being, a human person.

P2 (Death): Death is organic death.

The death of the human subject is his or her organic death, i.e. the end of his or her organic life.

P2 (Conception): Life is organic life.

The conception of a human subject is the beginning of the generation of his or her body, that is, the beginning of his or her organic bodily life.

P3 (Death): Death is the death of the organism as a whole.

The end of the life of a human subject is the death of the organism as a whole. In death the organism ceases to exist as a living whole, a living unit, 'an independent biological unit'.[33]

P3 (Conception): Conception is the beginning of the life of the organism as a whole.

The beginning of the organic life of a human subject is the beginning of the life of the organism as a whole. At conception the organism begins to exist as a living whole, a living unit, 'an independent biological unit'.

P4 (Death): Death is determined by physical (biological) criteria.

The end of the life of the organism as a whole is to be determined by physical criteria concerning the structure and function of the organism. These are empirically determinable; no other, extraneous considerations are required.

P4 (Conception): Conception is determined by physical (biological) criteria.

The beginning of the life of the organism as a whole is to be determined by physical criteria concerning the structure and function of the organism. These are empirically determinable; no other, extraneous considerations are required.

P5 (Death): Death is brought about by an irreversible physiological change breaking down organic unity and wholeness.

Death (the condition of being dead) is a state of the human organism brought about by an irreversible physiological change in the organism which has disintegrated (destroyed) its organic unity and wholeness. The cause of the disintegration can ultimately be traced to an irreversible loss of the brain's structure without which the organism cannot live.

P5 (Conception): Conception is brought about by an irreversible physiological change giving rise to organic unity and wholeness.

Life (the condition of being alive) is a state of the human organism brought about by an irreversible physiological change, an event (fertilisation) which gives rise to the organism as an integrated living unity, a living whole. If no damage or interference occurs the organism continues to live as a unit, as an organic whole, to adulthood.

P6 (Death): Death comes about through a process.

The end of a human life comes about through a process of organic disintegration (cellular disintegration), which eventually destroys the unity of the human organism as a unit, as a whole.

P6 (Conception): Conception comes about through a process.

The beginning of a human life comes about through a process of organic integration (cellular fusion) which generates the human organism as a unit, as a whole.

P7 (Death): **Death is the end of a process and a natural event.**

The end of the process of disintegration of the organism as a whole, a natural event, is death. Death is not the process itself, but that which ensues from the process; it involves a substantial change from the living state to the 'dead state', from living organic existence to non-existence of the organism.

P7 (Conception): **Conception is the end of a process and a natural event.**

The end of the process of organic integration bringing into existence the organism as a whole, a natural event, is conception. Conception is not the process itself but that which results from the process. It involves a substantial change which is undergone by two living cells (ovum and sperm) through fertilisation; each of these cells previously constituted part of a living whole, but now each ceases to be a part, and together they become a new living whole; this substantial change is a change from the non-existence to the existence of the organism.

P8 (Death): **Organic criteria provide a universal standard for determining death.**

The end of the process of disintegration of the organism as a whole is determined and defined by non-arbitrary organic criteria. The determination of when that process is at an end is not a matter of arbitrary decision. The criteria, because they are empirical, are of universal significance, that is, they provide us with a universal standard for deciding whether or not death has taken place, applicable to every human being without distinction. The criteria can be understood and appreciated by ordinary people using their powers of perception and common sense, and can thus be incorporated in legal and medical codes.

P8 (Conception): **Organic criteria provide a universal standard for determining conception.**

The end of the organic process of cellular fusion at fertilisation which gives rise to the generation of the organism as a whole is determined and defined by non-arbitrary empirical criteria. The determination of when that process is at an end is not a matter of arbitrary decision. The criteria, because they are empirical, are of universal significance, that is, they provide us with a standard of determining that human conception has taken place which is applicable to the life of every human being. The criteria can be understood and appreciated by ordinary people using their powers of perception and common sense, and can thus be incorporated in legal and medical codes.

P9 (Death): **In death the self-sustaining power of the organism is lost; time and nourishment will not effect the recovery of that power.**

The death of a human subject occurs when his or her organism dies as a whole. His or her physiological make-up is so damaged, deficient or destroyed that its power to sustain itself as a living unit is no longer present: it is irreversibly lost because the brain is dead. To wait for recovery or to provide nourishment in these circumstances is pointless. (Clearly, the loss of the power of 'being in existence' as a living whole is the loss of all powers in the human being.)

P9 (Conception): **In conception the self-sustaining power of the organism emerges; time and nourishment will effect the continuity of that power.**

The beginning of the life of a human subject occurs when his or her organism is generated as a whole; his or her physiological make-up is such that it has the power of maintaining itself in existence as a living unit, and this power is present at all times. To wait and to provide nourishment and shelter in these circumstances is highly important and valuable for the preservation of the organism as a whole. (Clearly, the preservation of the power of continuing in existence as a living whole amounts to the preservation of all other powers of the human being which in time will become manifest.)

V. Three concluding remarks

35. By way of conclusion I want to make three brief points. First, I wish to stress that there is a need to re-examine the double standard currently in use to determine, on the one hand, what counts as a living human subject in the case of death, and, on the other hand, what counts as a living human subject in the case of conception. The arguments about brain-stem death presented above make this double standard manifest. For in judging that death has occurred we proceed both medically (clinically) and legally, basing our judgement on the organic criterion, that is, the criterion of the disintegration and ceasing-to-exist of the organism as a whole. This is not the criterion currently used in the case of conception. Our common humanity rests on the fact that we all share our bodily condition, we are all human organisms, we are all members of the same human family – the species *homo sapiens*. This membership rests on our human organic make-up.

36. Secondly, as the opening paragraph of this paper shows, the true view of death as brain death (defended by the medical profession as described above) is still poorly understood or even misunderstood. A responsible understanding of that criterion of death needs to be attained and appropriately represented and summarised in public debate. (See, for example, section 88 of the document *Personal Origins*, published by the Board of Social Responsibility of the General Synod of the Church of England in June 1985, where brain death is misleadingly considered to be the end of 'personal life', and not primarily the end of the life of a human being, of a human organism as a whole, that is, the end of the organic life of a person.)

37. Finally, most current discussions of what counts as a human subject at the beginning and end of life are really, and ultimately, discussions about the ethics of killing, that is, discussions about the justifications to be found so that some

human beings may engage in the killing of some other human beings who are either severely handicapped, demented, newly conceived or brain-damaged, or with some other bodily deficiency which is considered to provide grounds for denying them an absolute right to human care and justice. It should not be possible, at this stage of our civilisation, to accept that there are two classes of human beings: those who are persons and those who are non-persons, the latter class having the status of things, property or chattel – in other words, the status which slaves used to have in law and in the practice of their masters.

7

European Legislation on Questions Concerning Artificial Insemination: A Report to the European Parliament

INTRODUCTION

1. The field of my specialised expertise within philosophy is bioethics, and in particular the area of human generation. From my experience in this field I shall approach the moral evaluation of the 'questions concerning artificial insemination (*in vivo* and *in vitro*) and the subsequent stages leading to the birth of a child' (Terms of Reference, from the letter of invitation).

2. My discussion will be divided into three parts. First, I shall set out my understanding of artificial insemination, its fundamental human significance and some of its concrete aspects. Secondly, I shall be concerned with the moral dimensions of the questions that artificial insemination raises, and, in accordance with indications found in the Working Document sent to me, I shall present 'a preliminary determination of the criteria for assessing the problems connected with artificial insemination' (p. 9). Thirdly, I shall deal with a fundamental question which underlies most of the ethical problems connected with artificial insemination. The question is formulated in the Working Document in the following terms: 'When does the life of a human being begin?'. Another way of framing this question would be: 'Does the beginning and the end of the organic bodily life of a human being constitute the beginning and the end of his or her human existence?' As a summary some conclusions will be presented.

PART ONE

I. The essential significance of artificial insemination

3. Scientific knowledge and techniques have made it possible to isolate, culture, mature and maintain alive for a period of time the ovum and the sperm cells outside a man's or a woman's body. (By a process of freezing, cells may be kept alive latently for an indefinite period of time.) As a consequence, the mature ovum and sperm may be brought together by technical intervention so that the process of their fusion (fertilisation) may occur. Therefore by these means fertilisation may be attained outside the human body (*in vitro*) or inside the human body (*in vivo*), or in some other host animal womb. This is the actual background which explains how the expression 'artificial insemination' refers to a process of technical intervention that brings together ovum and sperm cells with the aim that fertilisation may occur.

(i) The child newly conceived

4. The ultimate significance of the reality of bringing ovum and sperm together lies not merely in the technical means used but in the reality aimed at. It is intended that artificial insemination be followed by fertilisation, whereby an embryo is formed, the life of a new being, a member of the human species, begins; or, put in ordinary human terms, a child is conceived. The report of the Ethics Committee of the Royal College of Obstetricians and Gynaecologists on *In Vitro Fertilization and Embryo Replacement or Transfer* (London, March 1983) acknowledged this fact in the following terms: Doctors and scientists 'are taking part in the formation of the embryo itself. That role brings a special sense of responsibility for the welfare of the child thus conceived' (Section 6:1).

5. If artificial insemination did not give rise to fertilisation, and if in fertilisation (whether in the human species or any other mammalian species) we failed to recognise that a new individual of the species was conceived and began the course of his or her life, we would not be gathered here today. Governments and parliaments would not be concerned with how to enact

legislation regarding the protection due to the human embryo if this newly-conceived being were not of special human significance. This is the case regardless of what words are used to name or describe this new being, whether the word chosen is 'embryo', 'pre-embryo', 'not a full human', 'a biological process', 'a cluster of cells', 'a human biological node', 'human tissue', 'human genetic material', 'a potential human', 'the product of conception', 'a conceptus', 'a blob of cells', etc. The new being is indeed a newly-conceived human being, that given time and nurture will grow of itself into the adult being. The law of its organic finality is dynamically written within itself at every stage of its existence from the moment that the process of fertilisation is completed and it has the formation of a conceptus. Our problems do not lie with what embryology books clearly describe; embryological facts need not be distorted.

(ii) Human parenting

6. A child is conceived as the result of the actions of persons, and comes into the world within a community of persons. These persons carry out decisions and exercise responsibilities towards the care of the newly conceived and born child which constitute the context of what we understand to be human parenting or parental care. In every act of human generation human persons are always involved:

(a) persons (male and female) from whose gametes or cells the new being is generated;

(b) persons whose actions make possible that generation, and the gestation of the child;

(c) persons assuming responsibilities for the care and nurture appropriate to the different stages of growth of the child until it matures in all its human dimensions.

7. We regard as parents those two persons involved in conceiving, gestating and caring for the newborn infant with a total and unified responsibility. They are a father and a mother who, in mutual commitment to each other and to their offspring, constitute a community of persons, the family. The family is widely recognised to be, from every point of view,

the ideal type of community of persons in which human parenting, and so the wholeness of growth of the new child, can take place. It is not a credit to our contemporary mode of living and of relating to one another that we have appalling statistics of child suffering and child destruction at the hands of human adults, as a result of a breakdown of family life and family relationships (cf., e.g., statistics in England at present).

8. With the advent of artificial insemination the parental responsibilities of persons involved in (a), (b) and (c) above can now be separated and dissociated from one another and combined in a variety of ways with the aid of technical intervention. Parents need no longer be two in number. The new techniques have given rise (i) to a variety of modes of human conception and gestation, and (ii) to a variety of modes of human parenting (see below, para. 22). Yet in the design of nature, human conception and human parenting are inseparably connected. For the newly-conceived and newly-born child necessarily requires parental care not only for its existence and survival, but also for the development of its total humanity in wholeness and integrity.

9. Thus, the fundamental issues that arise from artificial insemination hinge on our recognition that a human being is involved and consequently that we have obligations to this new being – obligations which are
(i) related to the child when newly conceived; and
(ii) related to the child as needing care for its development.
In this light, the question of human fertility and other related questions legitimately concern Parliament and the various committees of concerned organisations only in so far as they involve decisions concerned with the well-being of the child. No-one would reasonably oppose or interfere with the provision of assistance (medical or otherwise) to alleviate human infertility if the welfare of the child as described in (i) and (ii) above were not at stake.

II. Human conception following technical interventions

10. *LTOT (Low Tubal Ovum Transfer)*. By the use of laparoscopy, ova are aspirated from the follicles in the ovaries and

transferred to the tube near the uterus or to the uterus itself. Thus, the sperm can reach the ovum there by means of natural intercourse (or, by another form of sperm penetration, into the female genital tract). Fertilisation naturally occurs in the womb. This medical procedure has been in use at St Elisabeth Medical Center, Ohio, USA, since 1983; the first attempts to use this procedure were made in England by Ian Craft. (Cf. I Craft *et al.*, 'Human pregnancy following oocyte and sperm transfer to the uterus', *The Lancet*, 1982, i, pp. 1031–1033.)

11. *GIFT (Gamete Intra-Fallopian Transfer).* Once ova have been collected by laparoscopy and the sperm obtained, ovum and sperm are placed in a catheter and both cells transferred to the fallopian tube (to the site where fertilisation normally occurs); conception then takes place in the normal way. Twins have been born in England by this method. It is practised in the Department of Obstetrics and Gynaecology, University of Texas, San Antonio, USA. (Cf. R. H. Asch *et al.*, 'Pregnancy after translaparoscopic gamete intrafallopian transfer', *The Lancet*, 1984, ii, pp. 1034–1035.)

12. *AI (Artificial Insemination).* In this procedure, as commonly understood, semen from a man (the husband or another man) is introduced into the woman's genital tract via the vagina by some relatively simple technical procedure (there are even 'do-it-yourself' kits on the market). Fertilisation occurs in the natural way. This practice has been widespread clinically and non-clinically since the 1950s. (Cf. R. Snowden and G. D. Mitchell, *The Artificial Family: A Consideration of Artificial Insemination by Donor*, Unwin Books, London, 1981.)

13. *Lavage: Non-surgical ovum transfer.* Conception occurs in a woman after insemination is carried out with semen from the husband of another woman who will become the future recipient gestating mother. After five days of insemination, uterine lavage is performed on the ovum donor who has conceived. The recovered embryo is then transferred to the uterus of the recipient infertile woman. In January, 1984, an infant was born by this procedure, practised in the Department of Obstetrics and Gynaecology, Harbour-UCLA

Medical Center, Torrance, California. (Cf. J. E. Buster *et al.*, 'Non Surgical Ovum Transfer as a Treatment of Infertile Women: Report of Two Pregnancies', *The Lancet*, 1983, ii, pp. 223–224; M. Bustillo *et al.*, 'Non Surgical Ovum Transfer as a Treatment of Infertile Women', *Journal of the American Medical Association*, 1984, vol. 251, n. 9, pp. 1171–1173; see also pp. 1178–1181, ref. 'Legal Issues'.)

14. *Human Fertilisation in Host Animal Wombs.* Attempts to attain this mode of human conception, e.g., in a rhesus monkey and in sheep, are mentioned although not fully described in the literature. See R. G. Edwards, 'The Current Clinical and Ethical Situation of Human Conception *In Vitro*', in C. D. Carter (ed.), *Developments in Human Reproduction and their Eugenic, Ethical Implications*, Academic Press, London, 1983, p. 56; and C. Wood and A. Westmore, *Test Tube Conception*, Unwin, London, 1983, p. 45.)

15. *Human Conception in Vitro (IVF).* The practice of this mode of human conception began in the late 1950s and was carried out by research scientists as a scientific enterprise. In 1968 the first scientific team was formed in England. In 1978 the first baby conceived by this method was born. Now the practice of IVF has spread to most of the industrialised countries. In Britain alone there are thirty centres practising clinical human IVF and eight centres are concerned with experimentation on human embryos.

16. There is a difficulty in obtaining basic accurate numbers from the published literature concerning the practice and experimentations undertaken by each IVF team as regards (e.g.):
numbers of women (and men) treated,
numbers of embryos generated,
numbers of embryos transferred,
numbers of children born.
The IVF results or 'success rates' are usually given statistically and in percentages. Different statistics follow different criteria. Professor Carl Wood, one of the IVF pioneers in Australia, has stated that because the IVF technique is of such recent development and is developing so rapidly, 'the

important matter of success rates has been dealt with arbitrarily' (*Test Tube Conception*, 1983, p. 96). Nevertheless, there is a certain amount of agreement among the practitioners concerning the percentages involved in IVF success rates. These can be summarised as follows:

17. *Results of IVF reported in the scientific literature:*
(i) *90% embryo loss in IVF/ET* (ET = 'Embryo Transfer'); 10% embryo survival. Cf. A Lopata *et al.*, 'The potential of the human egg to produce viable embryos and pregnancies', in *Journal of In Vitro Fertilization and Embryo Transfer* (hereafter abbreviated JIVFET), 1:2, 1984, p. 122.
(ii) *96% embryo loss in IVF/ET if allied to cryopreservation.* (Cryopreservation is the freeze-thaw embryo procedure.) Cf. J. Fleming and T. Iglesias, 'Human fertilization *in vitro* compared with nature', *The Lancet*, i, 1985, p. 168. See also: Committee to Consider Social, Ethical and Legal Issues Arising from IVF, *Report of the Disposition of Embryos produced by IVF* (the Waller Report), Government of Victoria, Melbourne, 1984, pp. 1–10.
(iii) *50% embryos killed by the freeze-thaw technique.* Cf. L. R. Mohr and A. Trounson, 'Freezing and donation of human embryos', JIVFET, 1:3, 1984, p. 127; and 'Deep freezing and Transfer of Human Embryos', JIVFET, 2:1, 1985.
(iv) *60% embryos 'unviable' (i.e., of abnormal or deficient structure) after fertilisation in vitro.* See C. O'Neil and D. M. Saunders, 'Assessment of embryo quality', *The Lancet*, ii, 1984, p. 1035; also A. Trounson and A. H. Sathanathan, 'The application of electron microscopy in the evaluation of two- to four-cell human embryos after *in vitro* fertilization', JIVFET, 1:3, 1984, pp. 153–165.

18. The abnormalities of embryos reported are of various kinds. The two most significant ones are:
(i) *10% polyploid embryos.* These usually arise from polyspermic fertilisation, when there is a failure of the natural system of the mature ovum to block the entrance of more than one sperm. Cf. E. Rudak *et al.*, 'Chromosome analysis of human oocytes and embryos fertilized *in vitro*', JIVFET, 1:2, 1984, p. 135; M. Plachot and J. Mandelbaum, 'Impairment of

145

human embryo development following abnormal fertilization *in vitro*', JIVFET, *ibid.*, p. 131; S. Al-Hasani *et al.*, 'Frequency and possible causes of polyspermic fertilization in an *in vitro* programme', *ibid.*, p. 97.

(ii) *Embryos with chromosomal abnormalities.* Cf. R. R. Angell *et al.*, 'Chromosome abnormalities in human embryos after *in vitro* fertilisation', *Nature*, 303, 1983, pp. 336–338.

19. *Causes giving rise to abnormal embryos: inducement of multiple ovulation.* A variety of causes producing abnormal embryos are mentioned. The most significant one is the hormonal intake to induce multiple ovulation in the female. Multiple ovulation is used by every IVF team at present. It is known to have deleterious effects not only on the human ova but on the whole female hormonal system and the various organs controlled by it – e.g., ovaries, oviducts, uterus, cervical mucus, etc. Multiple ovulation is advantageous quantitatively but not qualitatively, for it produces a large number of ova which facilitate the procedure, but neither the ova nor the female organism are benefited by the procedure; on the contrary they are deleteriously affected. This procedure gives rise, of course, to 'spare embryos'.

20. *Infertility.* Originally the primary professed aim of IVF teams was to alleviate infertility in cases of tubal occlusion, although it is also used now for many other conditions. Ninety per cent of cases of tubal occlusion are caused by previous abortion, the use of the IUD as a contraceptive device and sexually transmitted diseases. (Cf. J. McLean's survey, University of Manchester, Department of Anatomy, 1984). Note also that 'Evidence is now accumulating to suggest that tubal infertility is often due to pelvic inflammatory disease caused by sexually transmitted infection'. (See 'Recommendations for Priority Areas in Human Reproduction Research 1984', by the European Council's Advisory Sub-Group on Human Reproduction, in *The Lancet*, June 2, 1984, pp. 1228–1230. This document illustrates clearly the direction taken by present studies in human reproduction, and is highly significant as coming from the European medical profession in this field. Note that no programme of preventing the causes of

infertility is envisaged; the indications seem to be to the contrary.)

21. *The case of Zoe.* Zoe is the first baby born after having been conceived by IVF and then frozen and thawed out as an embryo. (See, for example, the report in the *Sunday Times*, 28 March, 1984). The salient features of her case are as follows:
- A team of 12 people, led by Professor Carl Wood (Australia), made this possible;
- 11 eggs were taken from the mother after induced ovulation;
- 10 of these eggs were fertilised;
- 3 embryos were transferred to the mother immediately; they died;
- 6 embryos were frozen at −196°C;
- 1 embryo was discarded as unsuitable.

When the frozen embryos were thawed for a new transfer:
- 4 embryos were found damaged and unsuitable for transfer;
- 2 embryos were transferred to the mother when her cycle was normalised;
- 1 embryo developed: little Zoe, a normal baby girl, was born on 28 March, 1984.

PART TWO

III. Moral questions

22. With the advent of artificial insemination the following procedures have become possible:
- gamete and embryo donation, storage and purchase;
- embryo sexing (following experiments on animals);
- gamete and embryo manipulation and research both at the cellular and the molecular level;
- transfer of the newly-conceived embryos from glass dishes, or from host wombs.

A variety of possible forms of parenting follow from the separation and combination of (a) an ovum-mother, (b) a conceiving mother, (c) a gestating mother, (d) a sperm-father, (e) a gestation-caring father, (g) a newborn caring father, (h) a clinical care and/or social care team, etc.

However, a set of fundamental questions arise concerning:
(i) human conception; and
(ii) human parenting.
Among these questions are the following:
- Should human beings be conceived in the laboratory from 'anonymous' gametes, given that the latter are regarded as suitable objects for experimentation and are used as such?
- Should human beings be conceived (and gestated) in host animal wombs?
- Should 'spare' embryonic human beings be deliberately conceived?
- Should the newly-conceived be bought and sold and regarded as property?
- Should the gestation process of a child be 'hired' or paid for?
- Should a child be brought into existence with the intention that he or she will grow up with only one single parent (male or female)?
- Should children be denied knowledge of their parental origins?
- Should 'the right to have a child' of some human beings be implemented at the expense of the lives of others?

23. These questions are moral questions with far-reaching legal implications, since they are concerned with ways in which newly-conceived human beings come to be generated individually and to be introduced and established in society. The overall moral question that needs to be answered is one of fundamental justice: What recognition and treatment is due in justice to all human beings unconditionally, and so to the newly-conceived and to children? The overall legal question is this: Should the law permit and foster unjust treatment of human beings when they are newly-conceived, or of grown children, by depriving them of fundamental rights?

IV. Moral criteria

24. The moral criteria for answering the above questions centre on the value of the individual human being. A commitment to the good and progress of 'humanity' necessarily takes the concrete form of a commitment to the good and progress

of every individual human being. 'Humanity' is real in the concrete only as individual human beings. Ultimately, there are two possible evaluations of the individual human being: either he may be used, harmed, disposed of, exploited, destroyed for the benefit of another human being or he may not. Either he is treated as an end in itself (and not as a mere means) or he is not.

25. The recognition that every individual human being is of intrinsic and non-instrumental value is one which the human family has attained and manifested in its abolition of slavery for every human being, including children. It amounts to the recognition of the fundamental moral equality of all human beings, an equality which is based on their shared humanity. This recognition may be formulated in the principle: 'No human being is property'; for property may be bought and sold, it may be used and disposed of, rejected or accepted as a commodity, depending on its quality as a product. In the case of human slaves, the lives and liberty of human beings were disposable in the interests of their masters.

26. Recognising the equality of all human beings amounts to recognising the primacy of respect due to the two fundamental dimensions of their being: life and liberty (or 'conscience' as Amnesty International puts it). In 1948, for the first time in human history, many nations of the world united to acknowledge, in the Universal Declaration of Human Rights, the fundamental equality of each and every member of the human family. The Preamble to this Declaration talks of 'the right to life and liberty' of each person (Article 3), the prohibition of all forms of slavery (Article 4) and the demand that each person should act towards his fellow human being in a spirit of brotherhood (Article 1). Thus the nations of the world affirm in this document that the respect due to every innocent human being in his life, bodily integrity and conscience holds in every case. It is not conditional; the individual human being is of non-instrumental value.

27. This same moral vision is enshrined in other bills of rights, and in our laws which are designed to protect the individual

and to safeguard individual rights; it is central to the moral vision of the medical profession in its Hippocratic tradition, as expressed in the principle *Primum non nocere* ('First do not harm'); it is a cornerstone and first principle of traditional philosophies and wisdom of our whole Christian era; it is also the cornerstone of the moral life and thinking of religious traditions such as Judaism with its demand 'Thou shalt not kill' and of Christianity with its counsel of perfection to love one's own neighbour even to the point of giving one's life for him. It is unfortunate that this vision is not part of the modern utilitarian outlook, in which the life of the individual human being is regarded as a value that can be 'traded off' against other values.

V. The current trend: a fundamental principle of justice is being abandoned

28. The moral evaluation of the individual human being that underlies current trends in scientific-medical practice, and the whole ethical outlook manifest in these trends, rests on two basic presuppositions, namely:
(i) that the value and interests of science and the rest of society may override the value of the individual human being; and
(ii) that the newly-conceived human being does not enjoy full human status.
Let me give some examples of how various international associations, boards and committees are trying to change fundamental moral principles that are relevant to biomedical research by accepting (i) above, thereby abandoning a fundamental principle of justice.

29. The *Warnock Report*, published in Great Britain in 1984, professes to accept the general moral principle that the human being is an end in himself and should never be exploited by another human being; but it qualifies its acceptance of the principle by saying that it is true 'in almost every case'. Its actual words are: 'Even in compelling medical circumstances the danger of exploitation of one human being by another appears to the majority of us far to outweigh the potential

150

benefits, in almost every case. That people should treat others as means to their own ends, however desirable the consequences, must always be liable to moral objection' (8.17).

30. The *Proposed International Guidelines for Biomedical Research involving Human Subjects*, by CIOMS (Council for International Organisations of Medical Sciences, established under the auspices of the World Health Organisation and UNESCO) were drafted in order to update, maintain and circulate the particular ethical views adopted in the Declaration of Helsinki II. At the time the draft appeared I had the opportunity to send comments as a member of a bioethical centre. One of my statements was the following:

> The fundamental ethical spirit of 'Helsinki II' is lost in these *Proposed Guidelines*. In 'Helsinki II' primacy is always given to the benefits to be secured for the subject of research and this is never allowed to be overridden in the interests of science or society at large or particular social groups. This is not the case in the *Proposed Guidelines*. See the contrast between the following affirmations of the two documents:

> *Helsinki II* (1.5): 'Concern for the interests of the subject must always prevail over the interests of science and society'; (3.5) 'In research on man, the interest of science and society should never take precedence over considerations related to the well-being of the subject.'

> *Proposed Guidelines*: 'Children should in no circumstances be the subjects of research holding no potential benefit for them *unless* with the objective of elucidating physiological or pathological conditions peculiar to infancy and childhood' (Article 9); '[Pregnant and nursing women] should in no circumstances be the subjects of non-therapeutical research that carries any possibility of risk to the fetus or neonate, *unless* this is intended to elucidate problems of pregnancy and lactation' (Article 10; my emphasis).

> It is clear that in these cases (Articles 9 and 10) the exceptions to the general rule which are admitted give the social and scientific interests and benefits of research an importance which is allowed to override the interest and benefit of the individual subject. Thus it is my recommendation that the guidelines should be revised in order to make absolutely clear that in every instance of research (be it carried out on individual subjects or on whole communities), concern for the benefit of the individual person – or concern

151

that there should be no risk of harm for him or her – must always prevail over considerations relating to the interests of science and society or communities in society.

31. *The Declaration of Geneva,* which dates back to 1948, and which is a contemporary version of the Hippocratic Oath, demands of doctors the following commitment: 'I will maintain the utmost respect for human life from the time of conception'. In October 1983 the Assembly of the World Medical Association changed the Declaration so that it now reads: 'I will maintain the utmost respect for human life from the time of commencement.' It is argued that ' . . . precisely when and where life commences is left an open question', for – the medical commentator of *The Lancet* continues – 'embryos are not only being aborted, they are also being grown *in vitro . . .*' (*Lancet,* 10 December 1983, p. 1357).

32. The members of the International Advisory Board of the Third World Congress on *In Vitro* Fertilization and Embryo Transfer (Helsinki, 1984), in their statement on this procedure, accept experimentation on newly-conceived human beings up to the 25th day (section 10). Two members dissented from this section of the statement, one on the grounds that there is no scientific necessity for research on human embryos and that more animal studies are needed before such research could be scientifically justified. The statement asks (in section 12) for support from existing international agencies such as the World Health Organisation, the International Planned Parenthood Federation and the World Medical Council. (Cf. *Annals of the New York Academy of Sciences,* 442, 1985, pp. 571–572.)

33. Thus it should be noted that the principle that one may use, harm or destroy human beings as instruments in medical research is now accepted by some influential agencies and committees, not only for newly-conceived human beings but also for children and even adults. Others would maintain that the newly-conceived human is not a 'full' human being and that therefore its life and organic integrity need not be respected. The statement from the Third World Congress mentioned above puts it as follows: ' . . . human rights change

with increasing age, and there is no particular stage of human development when human life begins' (Section 8).

PART THREE

VI. Criteria for determining 'full humanness'

34. *When does the life of a human being begin?* From a biological point of view, the claim (often expressed in the words 'Life is continuous') that because a human organic life develops through various stages it is uncertain when the life of a human organism begins is simply untrue – as all embryology books testify. The recognition that the individual of the species has a clearly-specifiable beginning and end cannot be eliminated from biology in general or from developmental embryology in particular. Not to accept, or to attempt to cover up, the fact that living beings of the various species (including the human) are generated or come into being as individual organic wholes through fertilisation, that they develop and grow as wholes and die as wholes, is to fly in the face of all scientific evidence as well as common sense.

35. There are certain embryonic phenomena, such as mono-zygotic twinning, and the stages of totipotency and plasticity that characterise the cells of the early embryos, which, for some, constitute grounds for doubt as to whether the newly-conceived human being is really an individual or 'a full human being' until day 14 of development or some time later than that. In public debate these phenomena are not properly described, and the general impression given is that the early embryonic being is completely undifferentiated, that it is not a unique living whole through organic unification but a cluster of molecular elements or cells which are open to being brought into subsequent divisions and aggregations. The facts outlined in the following few paragraphs need to be kept in mind if this misleading and scientifically inaccurate picture is to be rectified.

36. *Established empirical facts of embryonic development.* Molecular differentiating activity in the cells of the newly-formed *conceptus* (both intra-cellular and inter-cellular) is present from

the beginning. Each embryo is always (i) of a differentiated kind of nature, that is, of a particular species with its own genetic individuality; and (ii) a centre of continuous differentiating molecular-cellular activity, leading to its full formation (Cf., e.g., D. J. Begley, J. A. Firth and J. R. S. Hoult, *Human Reproduction and Developmental Biology*, chapter 8, 'Embryogenesis and its Mechanisms', Macmillan, London, 1980, pp. 90–102.)

37. The totipotency of every individual cell of the early embryo, its ability to become a whole integrated being, is species-specific. It is present in the two-cell mouse embryo but lost when the two-cell stage is past (possibly this applies to the human embryo as well); it is present in the two-, four- and eight-cell sheep embryo but lost thereafter. This has been newly demonstrated in recent experiments on higher mammal species. (Cf., e.g., S. M. Willadsen and C. B. Fehilly, 'The development potential and regulatory capacity of blastomeres from two, four and eight-cell sheep embryos', in H. M. Beir and H. R. Lindner (eds), *Fertilization of the Human Egg in Vitro*, Springer-Verlag, Berlin, 1983, pp. 352–357.) In the human species the eight-cell stage of embryonic development occurs about 30 hours after fertilisation is completed: day 2 of life.

38. The fact that the *cells* of the early embryo can be disaggregated, aggregated and thus 'recombined' to form chimeric embryos is a manifestation of the regulatory capacity which embryonic living beings possess and which enables them (i) to make themselves whole again when they have been deprived of a substantial part of their organisms, and (ii) to assimilate or integrate molecular, cellular or even organ parts from other organisms. In other words, powers of 'grafting', 'transplantation', 'healing' and 'regeneration' are present in embryonic organisms.

39. This general idea concerning early embryonic development may be expressed in the following four statements:

(a) Living beings are organic wholes; as such they can shed parts (cells) which may become parts of other organisms.
(b) Living beings can shed parts (cells) which may become new

154

organic *wholes* themselves, either on their own or in combination with other parts.

(c) Living beings can be deprived of or damaged in substantial organic parts and yet regulate or regenerate themselves to continue to develop as well-functioning wholes.

(d) Living beings (of mammalian species) as whole beings neither divide from nor fuse with other whole beings, but their parts, which they can shed, can do so.

40. Thus, because living beings are organic wholes constituted of parts (molecules, cells, organs) they can be genetically and cellularly manipulated – they can be literally 'mixed up'; yet *this mixing up is not of living beings as wholes, or of whole living beings, but of their parts*. Every living being is individual, that is, organically individuated in all its dimensions from the time of its generation (whether this generation takes place sexually or asexually) until its death.

41. There are two rival sets of criteria in terms of which the newly-generated human organism, that is, the human *conceptus*, is said to be of full human status or not. For some, to be an organic or bodily being of human kind is not a sufficient criterion for being a full human being; other criteria must be met in order for a human being to count as truly human, e.g. the appearance of the nervous system, the possession of human bodily form at two months' development, self-consciousness, awareness of personal identity, coming to value one's own life, etc. In this approach what particular stage of development of the human being will be counted as relevant to guarantee humanness may vary from clinician to clinician and from school of thought to school of thought. This approach is inadequate because it is partial; it selects only certain features of the humanness of the members of the human species, dividing them into two categories: the 'lesser human' and the 'full human'. A partial criterion could have no universal significance, and 'human equality' would become a euphemistic and arbitrary expression with no definite meaning.

42. The second possible criterion for determining true humanness is based on the simple affirmation that the total reality of

155

humanness is given in the very fact of *being a living bodily being of the human species*. With the reality of the living body the reality of being human in all its dimensions is present, and must be acknowledged and respected. There is nothing humanly-personally real about ourselves which is not present in the living bodies we are. To conceive a living human body is to conceive a living human being. In dealing with grown human beings clinicians (and the law) identify a human bodily being as a human being absolutely, as a human person, even if (e.g.) the dimension of self-consciousness is irreversibly lost. Every doctor knows, as we all do, that when the body of his or her patient dies, the patient is dead. In certifying death the doctor's criterion is the state of the body. No other, non-physical and extraneous considerations are required. The bodily criterion is the only reasonable and possible criterion in terms of which we regard a patient as humanly dead.

43. It is an abuse of the clinical understanding and determination of death as 'brain death' to claim that human death ensues when 'personal identity' or 'self-consciousness' is lost because the brain is dead, regardless of the state of the rest of the organism. What the new understanding of death as 'brain death' establishes is precisely that we know that the human organism as a whole is dead when the brain stem is dead; we know that if the brain stem is not functioning, the unity of the organism collapses so that breathing, blood circulation and heartbeat also stop. Hence it is the organic death of the body as a unified whole, as a living unified being, which is at stake in brain-stem death, and not merely the death of one of the body's organs or the loss of conscious personal identity. (Cf., e.g., C. Pallis, *ABC of Brain Stem Death*, BMA, London, 1983.)

44. It is clear that there is no comparable criterion for determining who counts as a living human being, a living human person, than the criterion by which we identify a living human body. To be a living human organism – a living human body – is the necessary and sufficient condition for being identified as a living human subject, a patient. That is why clinicians rightly claim that the end of the life of the organism as a whole

156

is to be determined by empirical organic or bodily criteria; no other extraneous considerations are required. Since a bodily criterion is used to determine the end of a human life, the same criterion must be acceptable for determining its beginning; there should be no double standard. For after all, our considerations concern the coming-into-existence (the beginning-to-live) and the going-out-of-existence (the ceasing-to-live) of the same kind of organic entity. It is in the living human body that our full and total humanity is given. It is in and through our bodies that we are the kind of persons we are. Our humanity is that which all members of the human family share in virtue of which they are all truly equal, and in virtue of which their life and integrity is to be equally respected. In this light, the question raised above, namely, 'Does the beginning and the end of the organic bodily life of a human being constitute the beginning and the end of his life?' is to be answered 'Yes'.

VII. Conclusions and recommendations

45. (1) The most basic moral issues that arise from artificial insemination hinge on our recognition that by means of this procedure the generation of a new human being takes place and that consequently we have obligations to this newly-generated being. These obligations are related (i) to the child as newly conceived, and (ii) to the child as needing care for its development. Thus, the question of infertility and other related questions are the proper concern of legislators and those responsible for the formation of public policy in so far as they involve decisions connected with the well-being of the child in relation to its conception and parental care.

Some defend the proposition that the newly-conceived human being may be used, harmed and destroyed as a means to beneficial ends or as object of experimentation; some maintain that the newly-conceived human being is not human in the full sense; some believe that since every adult has the right to a child there are no particular forms of human parenting that should be given moral or legal preference to others. My response to these claims is summed up in what follows; it is based on the recognition that there must be fundamental principles of moral justice underlying any

157

decisions concerning public policy envisaged for the protection of the individual and the good of the community.

(2) The fundamental moral equality of all human beings is based on their shared humanity; the fact that each and every one of them is a member of the human family, or that (in biological terms) each one is a member of the human species. To be a member of the species *homo sapiens* is the necessary and sufficient condition for being identified as a living human subject, as 'one of us'. For it is in and through our living bodies that our full and total humanity is given; it is in and through our living organisms that we are the specific kind of persons we are. There is nothing real about ourselves that is not given in the living organisms we are. To dissociate 'full humanity' from our bodily condition, from the kind of organisms we are from conception to death would amount to a manoeuvre which divides the human family into the protected and the exploited, a division on which all forms of gross injustice rely.

(3) Laws are about establishing and implementing, socially, principles of justice. One of these principles enshrined in our laws is that the human bodily being is not property, not chattel; it cannot be bought or sold. To abolish this principle from present legal frameworks, and to introduce its opposite, is to accept and legalise a new form of slavery and so to deny the most fundamental requirements of a just society.

(4) A related principle of justice enshrined in our criminal law is that of the inviolability of every innocent human being. This is a principle based on the recognition of the intrinsic, non-instrumental worth of the individual human being. To introduce in law a new principle which denies the intrinsic worth of every individual human being will amount to upholding the view that some people (the most powerful) can use, harm, exploit and destroy others for their own benefit. The abortion law in Great Britain, for example, does not abolish the general principle of respect for the life of the innocent human being; rather the law explicitly states that abortion, in the cases permitted, is an exceptional situation in relation to the general principle. Yet if the general principle is

changed one will have thereby removed recognition of the value of every individual as a principle of law. If the fundamental rights to life, bodily integrity and conscience of the individual human person are not safeguarded and preserved by law, what will be preserved?

(5) As regards determining public policy concerning human parenting, justice for the child cannot be ignored. Society should not countenance procedures which deliberately set out to generate children in a free-for-all fashion and thereby deprive them of the natural family context in which their identity, integrity, individuality, sense of responsibility and sense of belonging are best promoted. There cannot be any social criterion to identify the just and proper context for procreation other than legally recognised marriage.

(6) It is also an injustice towards the child to make legal provision for deliberately depriving it of the opportunity of coming to know who its biological parents are. Children who are adopted (e.g., in England) are not deprived of this right.

Notes

Introduction: The in vitro conceptus and justice

1 A discussion and defence of these aims was made in 1981 at Bourn Hall Clinic (Cambridgeshire, England) when authorities on IVF from Great Britain, Switzerland, West Germany, Australia, USA, France and Austria gathered together. The proceedings of this gathering were published in *Human Conception In Vitro: Proceedings of the First Bourn Hall Meeting*, ed. R. G. Edwards and J. M. Purdy, Academic Press, London, 1982. (See Chapter 2 of this book, para. 4.) The destruction of embryos for therapeutic and scientific aims were also defended by a standing committee of the Joint European Medical Research Councils in 1983 (*The Lancet*, 19 November 1983, p. 1187.) In Great Britain the same position was taken by the majority of signatories to the Warnock Report in 1984. The main recommendations of this report formed the basis of the legislation approved by the British Parliament in 1990.
2 R. G. Edwards's own term; see *Human Conception In Vitro*, 1982, p. 373.
3 *Ibid.*, p. 263.
4 The aim of developing contraceptives/abortifacients using human embryos was envisaged over 20 years ago. This aim is still defended and forms part of current research programmes. See, e.g., P. Braude, M. Johnson and J. Aitken, 'Benefits of In-Vitro Fertilization', in *The Lancet*, 2, December 1989, p. 1329. See also the following note (5).
5 The 14th annual report of the World Health Organisation Special Programme's Task Force on Vaccines for Fertility Regulation, 1985, states that 'The embryo represents an ideal target for attack since it comes into contact with the maternal circulation at a very early stage in its development (p. 54). The same WHO task force is managing the development of the Anti-HCG hormone (anti-implantation vaccine). About this, Professor Warren Jones has said: 'The vaccination could . . . prove to be extremely effective in solving the problems of birth control in developing countries. The vaccination principle is very attractive . . . they have already been introduced to vaccines and they know that it is "good medicine"'; cf. *Interpharma Healthfile*, December 1986, p. 3. As far back as 1968, Professor R. V. Short of the Department of Veterinary

Clinical Studies, University of Cambridge (who later headed the IVF Scientific Unit at Monash University, Australia, and is at present in the Department of Physiology and Anatomy at Monash) stated: 'If we are to control human population one of the things we need to control is the human corpus luteum', cf. Ciba Foundation, *Foetal Autonomy*, Churchill, London, 1969, p. 6. The corpus luteum develops in the ovary and ensures, by its hormonal release, that the embryo continues to live and grow following implantation. If the functioning of the corpus luteum were to be cut off, the embryo could not continue its implantation stage in the womb and would therefore die. The role that IVF is playing in providing human embryos for testing anti-birth vaccines, including RU 486, whose alleged safety has been questioned (*Nature*, 16 April, 1987, p. 648), is not well publicised. Scientists in France had protested at the amount of misleading information related to IVF. In an article in *Le Monde*, December 18, 1987, 'Procreation and Disinformation', a compilation of facts on IVF made by scientists, including the IVF pioneer in France, J. Testart, states that these techniques have been 'the subject of disinformation without precedent in the field of human fertility'. (My thanks are due to Dr P. Norris for providing me with her publication on *In Vitro Fertilization and Population Control*, The Medical Education Trust, Liverpool, 1989, which contains this and further information about these matters.)

6 See, e.g., 'Are In-Vitro Fertilization and Embryo Transfer of Benefit to All?', by M. G. Wagner and P. A. St Clair, *The Lancet*, 28 October 1989, pp. 1027–1030.

7 At the time of writing (the middle of 1990), Bills related to the human embryo have been debated and passed, for example, in Britain and Germany – in the former permitting human embryo experimentation up the the 14th day of development, in the latter prohibiting it. Court cases related to IVF also show the centrality of this issue.

8 This is a view of justice usually ignored in discussions of justice in medico-ethical contexts nowadays. The 'principle of justice' which is often invoked in these contexts refers to distributive justice in relation to allocation of resources. Nevertheless the concept of 'attributive' justice is important because it lays bare the most fundamental claims of justice that human beings possess in virtue of what they are. See, e.g., P. Tillich's discussion of this concept in *Love, Power and Justice*, OUP, Oxford, 1977.

9 See, e.g., M. C. Cornel, L. P. Ten Kate and G. J. Te Meerman, 'Ovulation Induction, In-Vitro Fertilization and Neural Tubes Defects', in *The Lancet*, 23/30 December, 1989, p. 1530.

10 All those who defend the destruction of embryos must ultimately adhere to this view. P. Singer and D. Wells explicitly state it: 'We suggest that the embryo be regarded as a thing . . .' (Singer and Wells, *The Reproduction Revolution*, OUP, Oxford, 1984, p. 98). More recently similar views have been put forward by (e.g.) John A. Robertson in 'Resolving Disputes over Frozen Embryos', in *Hastings Center Report*, November/December 1989, pp. 7–11.

11 See, e.g., G. A. Annas, 'A French Homunculus in a Tennessee Court', in *Hastings Center Report*, November/December 1989, pp. 20–22. Earlier, in 1984 in Britain, the signatories to the Warnock Report stated (section 11.17): 'We recommend that the embryo of the human species should be afforded some protection in law'. (Three of the signatories of the Report did not subscribe to this view and demanded full protection.)
12 R. G. Edwards, *The Beginnings of Human Life*, Carolina Biology Reader, 1981, p. 3.
13 Quoted in Peter Gwynne, 'Was the Birth of Louise Brown only a Happy Accident?', *Science Digest*, October 1978, pp. 7–12.
14 L. Kass, *Towards a More Natural Science*, The Free Press, Glencoe, U.S.A., 1985, p. 105.
15 Words of Baroness Warnock, pronounced during an interview on the radio programme 'Morning Ireland', RTE, Dublin, 24 April 1990.

1. A basic ethic for man's well-being

1 A fuller account of the attitudes proper to the conscientious person may be found in P. K. Bastable, *The Person of Conscience*, Philosophical Studies Monograph, University College, Dublin, 1986. I am very much indebted to the author of this work for my views in this section and for the general perspective of my paper.
2 Carl Wood and Ann Westmore, *Test-Tube Conception*, George Allen & Unwin, London, 1983, p. 45.
3 An illustration of this claim may be derived from the evidence submitted by the British Royal College of General Practitioners (18 March, 1983) to the British Government's Committee of Inquiry into Human Fertilisation and Embryology (1982), as compared with the evidence submitted to the committee by other medical bodies.
4 Cf. 'Oral contraceptives and cervical cancer', in *The Lancet*, 10 December, 1983, pp. 1358–1359.
5 Cf. J. Rock and M. F. Menkin, in *Science* 100, 1944, pp. 105–107; and M. F. Menkin and J. Rock, in *American Journal of Obstetrics and Gynaecology*, 55, 1948, pp. 440–452.
6 Cf. R. E. Fowler and R. G. Edwards, 'Induction of superovulation and pregnancy in mature mice by gonadotrophins', in *Journal of Endocrinology* 15, 1957, pp. 374–384; and R. G. Edwards, 'Meiosis in ovarian oocytes of adult mammals', in *Nature* 196, 1965, pp. 349–351.
7 Cf. R. G. Edwards, 'Maturation *in vitro* of mouse, sheep, cow, pig, rhesus monkey and human ovarian oocytes', in *Nature* 208, 1965; and 'Maturation *in vitro* of human ovarian oocytes', in *The Lancet*, ii, 1965, pp. 926–929.
8 R. G. Edwards, 'The Current Clinical and Ethical Situation of Human Conception *in Vitro*', in C. D. Carter (ed.), *Developments in Human Reproduction and their Eugenic, Ethical Implications*, Academic Press, London, 1983, p. 56.
9 *Ibid.*, p. 5.

10 Cf. R. G. Edwards and C. P. Steptoe, 'Current Status of In-Vitro Fertilisation and Implantation of Human Embryos', in *The Lancet*, 3 December, 1983, pp. 1265–1269.

11 Cf. Ian Craft *et al.*, 'Success of Fertility, Embryo Number and In-Vitro Fertilisation', in *The Lancet*, 31 March, 1984, p. 732.

12 See (8) above, p. 78.

13 Cf. James Le Fanu, 'The Scientific Case against Embryo Research', in *Medical News*, 28 June, 1984, pp. 14–15. Also, it is noteworthy that the discovery of the genetic cause of Down's syndrome by Professor J. Lejeune was achieved without experimentation on human embryos.

14 The committee set up by the British Government in 1982, chaired by Dame Mary Warnock, to inquire into human fertilisation and embryology, produced a report, published 18 July 1984. On the basis of the report there was ongoing public debate which was followed by legislation approved in 1990. (See Introduction, para. 22.)

15 R. G. Edwards, 'The Case for Studying Human Embryos and their Constituent Tissues In Vitro', in R. G. Edwards and J. Purdy (eds.), *Human Conception In Vitro*, Academic Press, London, 1982, p. 372.

16 Most of the pro-life submissions, including five from different Catholic bodies, have adopted this position.

17 R. G. Edwards, in (8) above, p. 70.

18 Cf. *The Times*, letter to the editor on 'Decisions on Ethics and Embryos' by R. G. Edwards and P. C. Steptoe, 6 June 1984.

19 *Report of the Royal College of Obstetricians and Gynaecologists' Ethics Committee on In-Vitro Fertilisation and Embryo Replacement or Transfer*, London, March 1983, section 10.7.

An acknowledgement of gratitude is due to the editor of *The Tablet* for allowing me to use in this chapter material already published in his journal.

2. IVF: Ethical issues and social implications

I wish to express my gratitude to Professor J. M. Finnis and to Mr Luke Gormally, my colleague at the Linacre Centre, London, for having read this paper and for making valuable suggestions for its improvement. The views expressed here should not, of course, be attributed to anyone other than myself.

1 The Committee of Inquiry into Human Fertilisation and Embryology, established by the British Government in the autumn of 1982 under the chairmanship of Mrs Mary Warnock, had the following terms of reference:. 'to consider recent and potential developments in medicine and science related to human fertilisation and embryology; to consider what policies and safeguards should be applied, including consideration of the social, ethical and legal implications of their developments, and to make recommendations.' This report formed the basis of the legislation approved in 1990.

2 The Report of the Ethics Committee of the RCOG on IVF has also adopted some of the fundamental opinions of Dr Edwards, who presented oral evidence to the Committee: see the Report's Acknowledgements. See also the 'Helsinki Statement on Human *In Vitro* Fertilization', in *Annals of the New York Academy of Sciences*, 442 (1984), pp. 571–572.

3 R. G. Edwards, 'Reproduction: Chance and Choice', in D. Paterson (ed.), *Genetic Engineering*, BBC Publications, London, 1969.

4 *Ibid.*, p. 29. It is there said: 'Can we, for example, immunise people so that fertilisation or implantation are prevented?'

5 *Ibid.*, p. 28.

6 *Ibid.*

7 See F. O'Connor, 'Pluralism: Justice or the Interests of the Stronger?', in *Abortion and Law*, Dominican Publications, Dublin, 1983. The theme treated here is developed by O'Connor in relation to moral pluralism.

8 To my knowledge those who have raised and discussed this ethical question have been P. Ramsey, L. Kass and H. O. Teifel.

9 R. G. Edwards and J. M. Purdy (eds.), *Human Conception in Vitro*, Proceedings of the First Bourn Hall Meeting, Academic Press, London, 1982, p. vii.

10 A reading of (e.g.) Edwards and Purdy, *Human Conception In Vitro* (note 9, above), shows how many of the scientific aspects of human embryology related to IVF programmes were still unknown at that time (1982), and how many procedures still remained at an experimental level. This is the case even today.

11 R. G. Edwards, *Conception in the Human Female*, Academic Press, London, 1980.

12 Cf. Report 'Pregnancy from frozen embryo', in *The Times*, May 1983, by T. Duboudin in Melbourne.

13 Cf. (9) above, pp. 219–233; also R. G. Edwards and P. Steptoe, 'Pregnancy in an infertile patient after transfer of an embryo fertilised *in vitro*', letter in *British Medical Journal* 286, 1983, p. 1351.

14 See (9) above.

15 *Ibid.*, p. 380.

16 *Ibid.*, p. 384.

17 *Ibid.*, p. 380.

18 *Ibid.*, p. 363.

19 Cf. H. O. Teifel, 1982, 'Human In Vitro Fertilisation', in *The Journal of the American Medical Association* 247, 1982, pp. 3235–3243; also L. Kass, *The Ethical Dimensions of In Vitro Fertilization*, American Enterprise Institute for Public Policy Research, Washington, DC, 1978, and 'Implications of Prenatal Diagnosis for the Human Right to Life' (1973), reprinted in T. A. Mappes and J. S. Zembaty (eds.), *Biomedical Ethics*, McGraw-Hill, New York, 1981.

20 R. G. Edwards and D. J. Sharp, 'Social Values and Research in Human Embryology', in *Nature* 231, 1971, pp. 87–90.

21 *Declaration of Helsinki: Recommendations guiding medical doctors in biomedical research involving human subjects*, adopted by the 18th World Medical Assembly, Helsinki, Finland, 1964, as revised by the 29th World Medical Assembly, Tokyo, Japan, 1979, section I.5.

22 *Ibid.*, section III.4.
23 This point is shown in a masterly fashion in G. E. M. Anscombe, 'Modern Moral Philosophy' (1958), reprinted in G. E. M. Anscombe, *Collected Philosophical Papers, Vol. III: Ethics, Religion and Politics*, Blackwell, Oxford, 1981.
24 Francois Jacob (Nobel Prizewinner in Medicine 1965), *The Logic of Life: A History of Heredity*, translated from the French by B. E. Spillman, Pantheon Books, New York, 1973, p. 313.
25 Scientists for Life, *The Position of Modern Science on the Beginning of Human Life*, Sun Life, Greystone, Virginia, U.S.A., 1975, p. 8.
26 J. Lejeune *et al.*, *The Beginning of Human Life*, Law and Medicine Series, AUL Inc., Chicago, 1981. Cf. also a letter to *The Times* (16 April, 1983) from the zoologist Dr C. B. Goodhart of Gonville and Caius College, Cambridge. Also, K. L. Moore, *Essentials of Human Embryology*, Blackwell Scientific Publications, Oxford, 1988.
27 M. I. Evans and A. O. Dixler, 'Human In Vitro Fertilisation', in *The Journal of the American Medical Association* 245, 1981, pp. 2324–2327.
28 W. A. W. Walters and P. Singer (eds.), *Test-Tube Babies. A guide to moral questions, present techniques and future possibilities*, Oxford University Press, Auckland, New Zealand, 1982, p. 61.
29 P. Ramsey, *Fabricated Man. The Ethics of Genetic Control*, Yale University Press, New Haven, U.S.A., 1970, p. 61.
30 Cf. (28) above, p. 60.
31 Cf. *British Medical Journal* 286, 1983, p. 1591.
32 *Declaration of Geneva* (amended 1968). This requirement is even demanded of doctors by the *Declaration of Oslo* 1970, on therapeutic abortion.
33 Cf. H. O. Teifel, 'Human In Vitro Fertilization' (no. 19 above), p. 3241.
34 Cf. J. Hughes-Onslow, 'Nine months to 1984', *The Spectator* 30 April, 1983, p. 16.
35 Cf. L. Kass, *The Ethical Dimensions of In Vitro Fertilization* (no. 19 above)
36 Royal College of Obstetricians and Gynaecologists (U.K.), *Report of the RCOG Ethics Committee on In Vitro Fertilisation and Embryo Replacement or Transfer*, March, 1983, section 11.
37 R. G. Edwards and D. J. Sharp, 'Social Values and Research in Human Embryology' (see no. 20 above), p. 87.
38 RCOG Ethics Committee Report on IVF (see no. 36 above), section 13.5.
39 Cf. British Medical Association, 'Interim Report on IVF', *British Medical Journal* 286, 1983, p. 1594.
40 P. Ramsey, 'On In Vitro Fertilization', Law and Medicine Series, AUL Inc., Chicago, 1980.
41 L. Kass, *The Ethical Dimensions of In Vitro Fertilization* (see no. 19 above). In his more recent publication 'Making Babies: the New Biology and the "Old" Morality', in *Towards a More Natural Science*, Free Press, Glencoe, U.S.A., 1985, pp. 53–55, Kass presents a modified view of the matter.
42 H. O. Teifel, 'Human In Vitro Fertilization' (see no. 19 above).
43 British Medical Association advice on 'Severely Malformed Infants' in the *British Medical Journal* 286, 14 May, 1983, p. 159.

44 P. Steptoe and R. G. Edwards, 'Pregnancy in an infertile patient after transfer of an embryo fertilised in vitro', letter in the *British Medical Journal* 286, 1983, p. 1351. This letter is an excellent illustration of the causes for fear that researchers have in relation to the possible implantation of abnormal embryos.

45 Cf. RCOG Ethics Committee report on IVF; also the report submitted to the Warnock Committee by the organisation Maternity Alliance, in *Maternity Alliance Bulletin*, March–April 1983, no. 9.

46 See R. Snowden and G. D. Mitchell, *The Artificial Family. A Consideration of Artificial Insemination by Donor*, Unwin Books, London, 1981.

47 See L. Kass, *The Ethical Dimensions of In Vitro Fertilization* and 'Making Babies: The New Biology and the "Old" Morality' (note 41 above).

48 Cf. R. G. Edwards, 'Reproduction: Chance and Choice' (note 3 above), p. 29.

49 Cf. Dr Tony Weaver's letter 'CND and Communism', in *The Times*, 3 May, 1983.

3. IVF: The basic issue

1 P. Singer and D. Wells, '*In vitro* fertilisation: the major issues' (with a comment by G. D. Mitchell and a response by Singer and Wells), in *Journal of Medical Ethics*, 9, 1983, 192–199.

2 W. Walters and P. Singer (eds.), *Test-Tube Babies*. OUP, Oxford, 1982, p. 60.

3 See, e.g., M. Tooley, 'Abortion and Infanticide', in M. Cohen, T. Nagel and T. Scanlon (eds.), *The Rights and Wrongs of Abortion*, Princeton: A Philosophy and Public Affairs Reader, 1974, p. 59.

4 J. Teichman, 'Wittgenstein on Persons and Human Beings', in *Royal Institute of Philosophy Lectures*, 7, 1972/1973, pp. 135–136.

5 Sir I. Jakobovits, 'Jewish medical ethics – a brief overview', in *Journal of Medical Ethics*, 9, 1983, p. 112.

6 R. G. Edwards and J. M. Purdy (eds.), *Human Conception in Vitro*, Academic Press, London, 1982, pp. 372–373.

7 *Report of the Royal College of Obstetricians and Gynaecologists Ethics Committee on In Vitro Fertilisation and Embryo Replacement or Transfer*, London, March 1983; see section 10.7.

4. The human being and the right not to be killed

1 See discussion of this topic in J. Teichman's 'The Concept of Person', in *Philosophy*, 60, 1985.

2 See, e.g., P. Singer, *Test-Tube Babies*, OUP, Oxford, 1984.

3 The definition of person was given by Boethius and critically commented on by Aquinas in the *Summa Theologiae* 1a, 30, 4.

4 The discussion follows M. Tooley's arguments as he presents them in 'Abortion and Infanticide', in M. Cohen, T. Nagel and T. Scanlon (eds.), *The Rights and Wrongs of Abortion*, Princeton University Press, 1974, pp 52–84. What is quoted in this section is taken from this article.

Tooley develops his views in a fuller form in his book *Abortion and Infanticide*, OUP, Oxford, 1983.
5 E.g., P. Singer.
6 Simone Weil, 'Personality', in *An Anthology*, Virago, London, 1986, p. 93.
7 *Euthanasia and Clinical Practice: Trends, Principles and Alternatives. The Report of a Working Party*. The Linacre Centre, London, 1982, p. 32.
8 Simone Weil, *Lectures in Philosophy*, ed. P. Winch, CUP, Cambridge, 1984, p. 203.
9 See the Linacre Centre report *Euthanasia and Clinical Practice*, p. 26.

5. What kind of being is the human embryo?

1 Michael Polanyi, *The Study of Man*, Chicago, 1985, pp. 61–62.
2 For discussion of the first see David Holbrook's 'Medical Ethics and the Potentiality of the Living Being', in *British Medical Journal* 291, 17 August 1985, pp. 458–462.
3 This statement is to be found in R. G. Edwards and J. Purdy (eds.), *Human Conception in Vitro*, London 1982, p. 354.
4 Andrew Huxley, in *New Scientist*, 11 April 1985, p. 2 (italics mine).
5 R. Descartes, *The Philosophical Writings*, Vol. II, trans. J. Cottingham, R. Stoothoff and D. Murdoch, Cambridge University Press, Cambridge, 1985, p. 18.
6 For a question similar in moral significance see (e.g.) Ethics Committee of the Royal College of Obstetricians and Gynaecologists, *Report on In Vitro Fertilisation and Embryo Replacement or Transfer*, London, March 1983. In Section 13.5 it is asked: 'at what point in the development of the embryo do we attribute to it the protection due to a human being?'
7 R. J. Berry, in *The Times*, 6 February 1980, col. 6, p. 15.
8 J. Mahoney, *Bioethics and Belief*, Sheed and Ward, London, 1984, p. 69.
9 *Ibid.*, p. 81.
10 'Tampering with the unborn child', an editorial in *The Economist*, 14 July 1984, pp. 13–14. It is important to note that not all scientific studies accept 50% embryo loss as a finally established figure. Cf. (e.g.) P. G. Whittaker, A. Tylor and T. Lind, 'Unsuspected Pregnancy Loss in Healthy Women', in *The Lancet*, 21 May 1983, pp. 1126–1127.
11 As in Mahoney, *Bioethics and Belief*, p. 100.
12 Cf. J. M. W. Slack, *From Egg to Embryo: Determinative Events in Early Development*, CUP, Cambridge, 1985, p. 166. This is a very thorough scientific study in experimental embryology, concerned with the first weeks of life with a view to understanding the biological mechanisms of 'how an egg becomes an animal'. The phenomenon of twinning is treated as one among other general properties of animal embryos, discernible in experimental conditions against the background of normal development. Those types of animals which in their early embryonic stages are capable of twinning by division of the embryo, namely, mammals, birds, amphibians, insects, are not considered by embryologists to be polyembryonic in nature (that is, containing a number of

167

individual embryonic beings in the early stages of embryonic life) as some contemporary theologians assume. The author states on pp. 218–219: 'Certain responses to experimental interference – such as adaptation of proportions to a change in size, or twinning following the division of the embryo – are very widespread but it is not known whether these similarities in behaviour reflect similar biochemistry and similar dynamics, different biochemistry with similar dynamics or merely similar categories in the mind of the investigator. We know nothing for certain about the biochemistry of regional specification but suspect that the full range of signals and responses may be very complex. We do not even know whether the phenomena can be explained in terms of small subsets of substances or whether a mathematical theory of the 'whole egg' is what is required ... We are left with the feeling that the models are of more use as an aid to clear thinking than as possible explanations of reality.'

13 This point, and the one which follows it, are well illustrated by the work of S. M. Willadesen and C. B. Fehily, presented in 'The development potential and regulatory capacity of blastomeres from two, four and eight-cell sheep embryos', in H. M. Beir and H. R. Lidner (eds.), *Fertilization of the Human Egg in Vitro*, Springer-Verlag, Berlin, 1983, pp. 352–357.

14 Cf. Recent embryology texts such as C. P. Wendell Smith and P. L. Williams, *Basic Human Embryology*, third edition, London, 1984, pp. 9–27. The importance of cytoplasmic activity and its relation to the nucleus in cells is demonstrated by experiments carried out on animal embryos regarding the transplantation of nuclei from the cells of (e.g.) 60-cell embryos to the cells of two- and four-cell embryos: see the works cited in notes (12) and (13) above.

15 G. G. Grisez, *The Way of the Lord Jesus: Christian Moral Principles*, Chicago, 1983, p. 7.

16 *Ibid.*, pp. 7–8.

17 *Didache, Precepts of the Via Vitae*. It is there said: 'You shall not kill the fetus by abortion, or destroy the infant already born'; see *Early Christian Writings*, Penguin, Harmondsworth, 1976, pp. 227–230.

18 See J. Connery, *Abortion: The Development of the Roman Catholic Perspective*, Loyola University Press, Chicago, 1977, Cf. also David Braine, *Medical Ethics and Human Life*, Palladio Press, Aberdeen, 1982, Appendix A: 'Early Christian Documents'.

19 Sacred Congregation for the Doctrine of the Faith, *Declaration on Procured Abortion*, in *Vatican Council II, More Post Concillar Documents* (ed.) A. Flannery, Dublin 1975, pp. 441–453, paragraph 7.

20 As in J. Connery, *Abortion: The Development of the Roman Catholic Perspective*, pp. 304–305.

21 J. H. Newman, *An Essay on the Development of Christian Doctrine*, ed. J. M. Cameron, Penguin, Harmondsworth, 1973 (reproduction of the 1845 edition): see chapter 1, 'On the Development of Ideas', pp. 93–147.

22 A comment made by R. J. Hennessey, editor and translator of volume 48 of St Thomas Aquinas's *Summa Theologiae* (ST), Part 3, Questions 1–6,

Blackfriars edition, Eyre and Spottiswoode, London, 1970. The author makes this comment in connection with ST, 3a, question 6, article 4; pp. 163–164 of volume 48.

23 Aquinas's statements are taken, both in the Latin version and in the English translation, from the *Summa Theologiae*, Blackfriars edition: Volume 11, edited and translated by Timothy Suttor; Volume 15, ed. and trans. M. J. Charlesworth; and Volume 48, ed. and trans. R. J. Hennessey.

24 I have made some changes that I thought were necessary in the English translation of this passage.

6. Death and the beginning of life

1 P. Singer and D. Wells, *The Reproduction Revolution: New Ways of Making Babies*, OUP, Oxford, 1984, p. 98.

2 Richard M. Zaner (ed.), *Death: Beyond Whole-Brain Criteria*, Kluwer Academic Publishers, Dordrecht, 1988. The quotation is taken from the publishers' leaflet advertising the publication.

3 Robert M. Veatch, 'Whole-Brain, Neocortical and Higher Brain Related Concepts', in Zaner (ed.), *Death: Beyond Whole-Brain Criteria*, Dordrect, p. 174.

4 Alexander M. Capron, 'The Report of the President's Commission on the Uniform Determination of Death Act', in Zaner (ed.), *Death: Beyond Whole-Brain Criteria*, Dordrect, pp. 167–168. A complete list of the States of the U.S.A. which have adopted laws (on the determination of death) based on cessation of total brain function is given in this article.

5 Cf. C. Pallis, *ABC of Brain Stem Death*, a British Medical Journal publication, London, 1983, p. 27.

6 I. M. Kennedy, 'The Kansas statute on death – an appraisal', in *The New England Journal of Medicine*, 285, 1971, pp. 946–950.

7 C. Pallis, *op. cit*, p. 4.

8 Cf., e.g., David R. Smith, 'Legal Issues Leading to the Notion of Neocortical Death', in Zaner (ed.), *Death: Beyond Whole-Brain Criteria*, Dordrect, pp. 11–1144.

9 President's Commission for the Study of Ethical Problems in Medicine and Biomedical and Behavioural Research, *Defining death: medical, legal and ethical issues in the determination of death*, U.S. Government Printing Office, Washington, D.C., 1981, p. 2.

10 Conference of Medical Royal Colleges and their faculties in the UK, 'Diagnosis of Death', in *British Medical Journal*, i, 1979, p. 3320.

11 'Memorandum on Brain Death', in *Irish Medical Journal*, 1, no. 1, 1988, pp. 42–45.

12 *Ibid.*, p. 54.

13 C. Pallis, 'Brain-stem Death: The Evolution of a Concept', in P. S. Morris (ed.), *Kidney Transplantation* (2nd edition), Giune and Stratton, Orlando, U.S.A., 1984, p. 101.

14 Dr D. W. Evans has written and publicly stated both in the UK and in Ireland that the brain cannot be truly and totally dead while there is still blood circulation in the brain, even if 'brain stem death has been

diagnosed. He contends also that the means used (that is, the tests carried out) to diagnose brain-stem death are inadequate, so that there remain 'untested functions in the brain stem at the time when . . . the whole of the brain stem is said to be dead' (from an RTE interview, Dublin, 17 May, 1988).

15 See Capron, 'The Report of the President's Commission on the Uniform Determination of Death Act', in Zaner (ed.), *Death: Beyond Whole-Brain Criteria*, p. 159.

16 See President's Commission, *Defining death: medical, legal and ethical issues in the determination of death*, p. 28.

17 See C. Pallis, *ABC of Brain Stem Death*, p. i.

18 *Ibid.*, p. 2.

19 *Ibid.*, p. 3.

20 See J. Bernat *et al.*, 'On the Definition and Criterion of Death', in *Annals of Internal Medicine*, 94, pp. 389–394.

21 This is also the view of (e.g.) Alexander Capron and Christopher Pallis, although it is criticised by (e.g.) R. M. Veatch; see Veatch, 'Whole-Brain, Neocortical and Higher Brain Related Concepts', in Zaner (ed.), *Death: Beyond Whole-Brain Criteria*, Dordrect, p. 178.

22 See President's Commission, *Defining death: medical, legal and ethical issues in the determination of death*, p. 33.

23 See C. Pallis, *ABC of Brain Stem Death*, p. 8.

24 Discussed and referred to by E. Gilson in *From Aristotle to Darwin and Back Again*, Sheed and Ward, London, 1984, p. 122.

25 This point of view is presented and further discussed by David Lamb in *Death, Brain Death and Ethics*, Croom Helm, London, 1985, pp. 70–82.

26 For the discussion of this point see A. Kenny, *Will, Freedom and Power*, Blackwell, Oxford, 1975.

27 *Ibid.*, Chapter 7.

28 See Cf. C. Pallis, *ABC of Brain Stem Death*, p. 2.

29 *Ibid.*, p. 3.

30 *Ibid.*, p. 2.

31 This is the view defended not only by C. Pallis but also by (e.g.) A. Capron and L. Kass.

32 It will be clear to the reader, in view of what has been said in previous chapters, that what I am saying here in no way amounts to a denial of the human being's immortality or a failure to recognise his or her eternal destiny. What I mean to say here is that the bodily existence of the human being (i.e. his or her unique mortal human condition, as we know this condition to be for everyone), undeniably begins with conception and ends with death.

33 C. Pallis's expression; see his 'Whole-brain death reconsidered – physiological facts and philosophy', in *Journal of Medical Ethics*, 9, 1983, p. 33.

Index

171

172

intra-uterine device (IUD) 38, 39, 49, 146

Jacob, F. 43
Jakobovits, Sir I 166
Jewish-Christian tradition 42, 61, 150
John Paul II, Pope 109
Johnson, M 160
Jones, H. W. 21, 92
Jones, W. 160
justice 1–6, 12–15, 41, 60, 80, 81, 83, 84, 148, 150, 157, 158, 159

Kant, I 42, 61
Kass, L. 8, 51, 164, 165, 170
Kennedy, I. M. 114, 169
Kenny, A. 128, 170
killing, wrongness of 41, 43, 47, 50, 68, 72–73, 76, 80–84, (*see also*: right not to be killed)

Lamb, D. 170
laparoscopy 48, 142, 143
lavage 143
Le Fanu, J. 163
Lejeune, J. xii, 55, 163
Linacre Centre 5
Locke, J. 63, 73, 75, 76
Lopata, A. 145
low tubal ovum transfer (LTOT) 142

Mahoney, J. 96, 167
Mandelbaum, J. 145
Marshall, J. 88, 90
McLaren, A. xii
McLean, J. xii
Medical Research Council 24, 45
Memorandum on the Diagnosis of Death (UK) 115
Memorandum on Brain Death (Ireland) 115
Menkin, M. F. 20

'mere biological life' 74, 78–79
mind, human 128
Mitchell, G. D. 57, 58, 143
Mohr, L. R. 145
morality 40–43, 46, 76–77, 82
multiple ovulation 146
murder 82–84

neocortex and brain death 114, 115, 130
nervous system, and human personhood 75
Newman, J. H. 102

O'Connor, F. 164
O'Neil, C. 145
Offences against the Person Act (1861) 2
organ donation 118
organic wholeness, human 121–124, 128, 129, 130, 136, 153, 154–155, 156

Pallis, C. xii, 115, 116, 119, 129, 130, 156, 169, 170
Paul, St 102
persons and human personhood, 7, 9, 27–28, 63–68, 72–75, 112, 156
philosophy 10, 25, 26, 101, 104, 139
Plachot, M. 145
Polanyi, M. 87
potentialities and powers, human 8–9, 11, 65–67, 74–75, 78–80, 122, 127–129
'pre-embryo' 85, 95, 141
President's Commission (USA) 111, 114, 169, 170
Purdy, J. 21, 160

Quinlan, K. 118

racialism 42

173

174